D0525208

Introduction to language pathology

For Randoph Quirk,
in his sixtieth year

DAVID CRYSTAL

INTRODUCTION TO LANGUAGE PATHOLOGY

SECOND EDITION

C W

COLE AND WHURR
LONDON AND NEW JERSEY

© Cole and Whurr Limited 1988

First published 1980 by
Edward Arnold (Publishers) Ltd
Second edition 1988 published by
Cole and Whurr Limited
19b Compton Terrace, London N1 2UN

British Library Cataloguing in Publication Data

Crystal, David
    Introduction to language pathology – 2nd edition
    1. Language disorders
    I. Title
    616.8′55   RC423

ISBN: 1 871381 10 X

Printed and bound in Great Britain by
Biddles Ltd, Guildford and King's Lynn

Contents

Preface

The 1970s have seen the study of communication disorders at an important transitional stage in its development. In Great Britain, a series of government reports has initiated entirely new attitudes towards several of the professions involved—to speech therapy (the Quirk Report, 1972), remedial language teaching in schools (the Bullock Report, 1975), and to the education of the handicapped (the Warnock Report, 1978). New degree courses at undergraduate and postgraduate levels have broadened the academic basis of training in the subject, and several new journals have appeared, reflecting these interdisciplinary connections. There have been considerable advances in investigative techniques, both in special instrumentation and in analytic procedures, which have produced enormous amounts of fresh data. But most of all, there has developed a new critical awareness of the limitations of the traditional categories, nomenclature and practices involved in the study of handicap in general, and of speech disorders in particular. The influence of such developments is undoubtedly fundamental, though it is by no means clear what shape will finally be given to the academic and clinical discipline currently being formed. Meanwhile, new terminology exists alongside the old; newly-trained therapists and teachers have to work alongside older-trained but more experienced colleagues; there is a persistent demand for collaboration between specialisms (in both clinical and teaching practice and in research). It is an intellectually stimulating and clinically rewarding time. But for the new student of the subject, or for the layman wishing to develop an awareness of the subject, the excitement and stimulation is often somewhat diminished, as he struggles to master the competing traditions, techniques and terminologies.

My aim in writing this book has been to reduce the confusion regularly admitted by people who encounter the field of communication disorders for the first time. The lack of orientating textbooks at first-year level is only too apparent. I have therefore tried to do two things: to provide a general view of the field which will enable the student to interrelate the main components of study; and to provide enough of an introductory account of each of these components to enable the student to see their role in clinical investigation. It has been an exercise in the old manner of trying to see both the wood and the trees simultaneously. But in a short book, something must give; and my hope is that the brevity with which many areas have been covered will be justified by the overall perspective which I have tried to achieve. The book has another deliberate bias. Several years of running a first-degree course in this field has brought home to me the unique problems posed by its multidisciplinary character. At Reading, we have a weekly 'bridging seminar' in which the aim is to juxtapose the contributory lecture courses and associated reading, and to focus on differences in theory, method and above all terminology which identify the various subjects. I have been repeatedly struck by the way in which apparently innocuous terms give rise to major problems of interpretation and attitude. I have therefore tried to anticipate terminological problems throughout this book, and explained all technical notions as they have arisen. While this procedure does slow the pace of the book in places, I am sure it is a desirable emphasis, in the present state of the field.

The other characteristic of this book is that I have adopted a relatively conservative approach to the subject. I have for the most part incorporated the traditional categories of classification in speech disorders, and contented myself with pointing out the main difficulties to which several of these categories give rise. Only in a very few cases have I gone so far as to recommend a usage, or the avoidance of a usage. Nor have I introduced as much of an orientation from clinical linguistics as I know will one day be needed. This would be premature, given the limited application of that subject to date; in view of its relatively undeveloped form, such an approach is best handled at monograph level (see my *Clinical linguistics* (1981/7)). The point is worth stressing, for I am anxious that readers who have encountered my previous work in linguistics will not expect from the present book too radical an orientation arising out of my background in that subject. The underlying philosophy of the book does reflect very largely what I have learned from linguistics, as will be apparent in several places. But many of the descriptive sections reflect no more than what I have learned from those disciplines with whom I have found myself collaborating increasingly in recent years. In general, I have tried to strike a balance between these influences—especially, between the classical medical concepts and the newer behavioural ones, as discussed in Chapter 2. I am in no doubt that, in the long term, it is the latter emphasis which will promote the development of the explicitly principled intervention procedures which language pathology so badly needs. For the present, I leave it to more advanced courses and textbooks to take further the implications of the linguistic orientation, when this becomes apparent throughout the book.

D.C.
1 August 1979

Preface to the second edition

I began the first edition of this book by commenting on the irony that the name of the subject of language disorders, and the associated profession, should be a matter of such dispute, at the time of writing. Nearly a decade has passed, a new edition is being prepared, and the matter, it seems, continues to rouse just as much emotion. Recent issues of the monthly bulletin of the American Speech-Language-Hearing Association, *Asha*, have carried a series of letters representing the whole spectrum of opinion. In August 1987, for example, we find a writer condemning 'pathologist' and 'language' and opting for 'speech therapist'; in January 1988 another writer considers such a change to be retrograde; but in February 1988 there is support expressed for the anti-pathologist position, the writer sharing the view that the term is a source of confusion in the minds of the public. Further contributions are to be expected. In Britain, too, the matter has been regularly raised in the 1980s, and has come to the fore again in the month I began to prepare this new edition. In the College of Speech Therapists Bulletin for April 1988, following another chain of correspondence on the topic, it was proposed that the whole matter should be referred for judgement to the new President of the College, Professor Sir Randolph Quirk who, as an expert in the English language, might be able to devise a suitable name. It would be nice if this particular issue could be solved *ex-cathedra*; but the history of language planning suggests otherwise. My feeling is that the debate over the name of the profession will be with us for a while yet, and I have therefore not rewritten my opening chapter, which seems as relevant today as it was a decade ago. *Plus ça change, plus c'est la même chose.*

And yet, things *have* changed. The 1980s has been a time of great movement in the field of language pathology, and in the lives of those professionals who work with it. When the time came for this book to be reprinted, therefore, it seemed essential to make a new edition, so that information about current issues could be introduced, and the facts updated about the many new books, tests, and journals which have developed from a trickle into a flood during the decade. In this second edition, therefore, an extra chapter on 'Current trends' has been written, the footnote references in all parts of the book have been radically revised, and the appendix on tests and assessments has nearly doubled in size, as has the section on further reading. I have also corrected a scattering of typographical errors and unclarities of exposition which found their way into the first edition. In this way, I hope that the book will maintain its relevance for those who will embark on their study of language pathology as we approach the new millenium.

D.C.
1 June 1988

Acknowledgements

A book of this kind betrays innumerable influences, all of which I would acknowledge, if only I could remember them. I know I gained a great deal from my membership of the Academic Board of the College of Speech Therapists over several years: colleagues there taught me a healthy respect for each of the contributing disciplines to this complex field. Successive generations of my language pathology students have, perhaps unwittingly, been an invaluable source of information about the problems that need to be tackled in writing about the field at an introductory level. There is no space to acknowledge the help I have had from my many academic, medical and therapist colleagues who have discussed their approaches with me; but I am specifically grateful to those who read through various drafts of this book and commented most helpfully on its content—John Bamford, David Chapman, Margaret Davison, Paul Fletcher, Mike Garman, Graham Ratcliffe, Marion Trim, Renata Whurr. For the second edition, I have benefitted from further comments received from Pamela Grunwell and John Connolly. And as always, the general support, advice and practical help I have found from my wife, Hilary, has been a major factor enabling the book to progress. It is my sincere hope that what I have learned from all these people is enough to ensure that the outcome will do no disservice to the patients and pupils whom they serve.

1

The scope of the subject

What's in a name? That which we call a rose
By any other name would smell as sweet.
   (*Romeo and Juliet*, II. ii.)

It is an unfortunate irony that the subject which professes to deal with the difficulties and disorders of language should itself be in difficulties over its name. But such is the case. One of the most awkward decisions encountered in planning this book was what to call it. Should we be talking about 'language pathology' or about 'speech therapy' or 'communication disorders' or 'remedial language problems' or . . .? The irony resides in the fact that it is only the title of the subject which is at issue. Each title carries different implications, as we shall see; but there is little real dispute as to what this subject of study actually consists of. The kinds of things that go on in speech clinics in the United States, under the supervision of people called 'speech pathologists', are very much the same as those that go on in the United Kingdom, under the supervision of people called 'speech therapists'. Likewise, on the continent of Europe, labels vary, but the job remains largely the same: in France, one is an 'orthophonist'; in Belgium and Germany, a 'logopaedist'; in Czechoslovakia, a 'phoniatrist' . . . What, then, is the job that all these people do?

All these people are professionals, trained to investigate and treat abnormal manifestations of language, for whatever cause, in children and adults. The skills involved are many, and take a three- or four-year training period to acquire. A rather fuller description is provided by the American Speech-Language-Hearing Association (the body which in the United States issues certificates of clinical competence to those who succeed in training). They expect their clinicians to have an 'in-depth knowledge of normal communicative processes, development and disorders thereof, evaluation procedures to assess the bases of such disorders, and clinical techniques that have been shown to improve or eradicate them' (1975 formulation). A recent textbook on the subject begins in a similar vein:

> As a diagnostician, the speech pathologist is a professional who (1) possesses a fund of knowledge relevant to speech and language disorders, (2) is skilled in applying this knowledge to solving clinical problems, and (3) has an overriding concern to helping a person, his client, understand and manage his speech or language problems.[1]

[1] J. E. Nation and D. M. Aram, *Diagnosis of speech and language disorders* (St. Louis, Mosby 1977),3.

The 1972 government report on speech therapy services in Great Britain gave an account of a similar range of skills, with perhaps greater emphasis on the relationship between speech therapy and other professions:

> The majority of our witnesses concurred in distinguishing, in the services offered by speech therapists, four elements: assessment, treatment, advice to patients and their families and an additional role, containing advice, teaching and the provision of information, in relation to teachers and members of other professions concerned with communication disorders.[2]

There is, it would seem, considerable agreement about what these professionals are doing—enough, at least, to suggest that a single name for the subject would not be a problem. Why is this not so?

The best way of explaining the problem is to focus on the implications of the term 'speech therapy', and the associated term 'speech therapist'. In the past ten years, these have been the subject of particular controversy in Great Britain. There are two main objections to these labels. Firstly, the profession does a great deal more than deal solely with speech. When there is a breakdown in a person's communicative abilities, it is often the case that much more than speech is affected. Other modes of communication can be involved, such as listening, reading, writing and signing. And even within speech, there is far more involved than the surface 'sound effect'. Beneath the surface lies a world of grammar and meaning, and this may also contribute to someone's problems in communication. 'Speech', in the view of many, is too restricting. Such people might prefer, instead, to talk about 'speech and hearing' therapy, or 'speech and language' therapy, or 'communication' therapy. There are obviously many possible permutations. The official journal of the British College of Speech Therapists is in fact called the *British Journal of Disorders of Communication*.

But if 'speech' causes problems, the term 'therapy' causes even more difficulty. This term is these days used in relation to a broad spectrum of activities, unrelated to its original sense of medical treatment. For example, it encompasses a whole range of personal and social problems, such as in 'community therapy', 'recreation therapy', and 'beauty therapy'. Many of these skills do not involve professional training of any kind, and those that do are often not comparable to the specialized academic training which speech therapists receive. As a consequence, many speech therapists fear that their status may be misleading, or be diminished in the eyes of the other professionals with whom they work. A particularly misleading implication, in their view, is that the term suggests that their only function is treatment—and moreover treatment under someone else's supervision. But this is far from being the case. Unlike most other 'paramedical professions' (that is, the many people who help to treat medical problems, but who are not doctors), speech therapists are the ones who are ultimately responsible for

---

[2] *Speech therapy services* (London, HMSO 1972), 57. The committee of enquiry was under the chairmanship of Professor Randolph Quirk, and is generally known as the 'Quirk Report'.

the diagnosis, as well as the management of their patients' linguistic disabilities. They do not work under the supervision of a colleague from a different discipline (such as a hospital consultant), and in this respect they are in a different category from, say, physiotherapists or occupational therapists. To fulfil their role, a whole process of investigation into the nature of the communication problems affecting their patients must take place before they may venture into therapy. It is plainly a highly responsible role, which (it can be argued) the term 'therapist' does not reflect, and which could prove to be misleading to other professionals, administrators, and above all to the public requiring their services.

These fears are not entirely well-founded, but they are nonetheless real. The medical notion of therapeutics, for example, is an extremely broad one, subsuming all aspects of patient management (including surgical, chemical, occupational and other kinds of treatment). If 'therapeutics' is felt to summarize well what physicians do, the analogous use of the term in the context of language disability might not be so misleading as is feared. Be this as it may, the objections to the label 'speech therapist' within the profession in fact became so strong that in 1973 the British College of Speech Therapists held a poll of its membership, to determine whether an alternative name might be found. In this poll, the membership was asked to choose between 21 alternative names that had been proposed. These were as follows:

communicologist	phasiologist
communication specialist	phraseologist
language pathologist	speech and language pathologist
language pathologist and therapist	and therapist
languologist	speech and language pathologist
linguologist	speech practitioner
logopaedist	speech and language therapist
oratologist	speech and language practitioner
ortholinguologist	speech pathologist
human communication specialist	speech pathologist and therapist
human communication practitioner	speech and language specialist

The results were inconclusive. No one label received an overwhelming majority. In fact, none of the alternatives proposed received as many votes as 'speech therapist'! Accordingly, a further vote took place (in 1974), the seven names receiving the largest number of votes being short-listed.[3] But again no decision was reached—indeed, only a small proportion of the membership voted the second time. It seemed that most of the alternatives had problems of their own. 'Logopaedist', for example, had a promising first element (suggesting language in general, and with medical connotations),

[3] The short list was 'speech and language therapist', 'speech and language specialist', 'speech and language pathologist', 'speech pathologist', 'speech pathologist and therapist', 'human communication specialist' and 'logopaedist'.

but a poor second element (suggesting children only, whereas a great deal of the speech therapist's work is with adults). Combinations such as 'speech and language pathologist and therapist' were felt to be too much of a mouthful—or eyeful (bearing in mind the need to fit the label onto a hospital lapel badge!). 'Languologist,' one person said, 'would be likely to cause more speech problems than cure them'! At the same time, there were some who argued that 'therapist' was perhaps not as bad a term as had been initially made out. It is self-evident that therapy presupposes other skills, it was said, and as it is by the results of their therapy that these professionals are judged, then the term should stay as the most convenient and familiar summary of the intentions of the profession. Faced with such a mass of conflicting opinion, the College's Council concluded at the time that the name should be unchanged, for the time being. But the matter was not dropped. Five years later, the question was raised again; further votes were taken, and the issue was finally reduced to a single choice: 'speech pathologist' v. 'speech therapist'. By the end of 1979, the matter was decided: a final vote resulted in a two-to-one majority in favour of 'speech therapist'.

Lest this should be thought to be a peculiarly British obsession, it should be pointed out that a similar concern has often been expressed in other countries where this profession is exercised. At present, also, there is a need to consider the merits of consistency throughout the world—throughout Europe, for example, in these days of the European Economic Community, or throughout the English-speaking world as a whole. Moreover, other professions have been faced with comparable terminological difficulties, as is illustrated by the debates over the labelling of children in the context of mental health or physical handicap,[4] or the discussion of the term 'remedial' in educational contexts. Nor is this terminological question trivial. What's in a name, indeed! The answer is: 'A great deal'. The issues involved are those of professional identity and status, academic orientation, intellectual, clinical and financial rewards.

This book, then, is not called an introduction to speech therapy, for two main reasons. Firstly, it makes no claims to provide guidelines for therapy. It could not, for its author is not a speech therapist. Secondly, it is about 'language' in all its forms, and not just about speech. The latter point is perhaps less controversial these days than it was, for reasons I shall go into below (p. 6). But the use of the term 'pathology' does still have its problems, which in the interests of clear thinking I must briefly discuss.

From the point of view of linguistic disability, the usefulness of the term 'pathology' is simultaneously its weakness—that it is a medical term, falling within a tradition where it is rigorously defined. One medical dictionary (Blakiston's) defines it as 'a branch of biological science which deals with the

---

[4] The government report on *Special educational needs* (the 'Warnock report', London, HMSO 1978), for example, illustrates the concern over terminology. One of their main recommendations is to get away from the tradition of labelling children as belonging to a specific category of handicap (such as 'educationally subnormal' or 'remedial'), replacing this by the notion of a scale of learning difficulties.

nature of disease, through study of its causes, its process, and its effects, together with the associated alterations of structure and function.' There are two central features of this definition for our purposes: it refers to 'disease', and this in turn refers to a disturbance of normal structure and function. In view of the fact that many of the conditions which speech clinicians treat are medical in origin, the result of disease, this alignment of their profession with the clinical world seems eminently sensible. On the other hand, by no means all of the conditions which are treated in a speech clinic are medical in origin, in any clear sense. A patient may have an apparently normal physical structure and function, as far as his vocal apparatus is concerned, and yet, for example, speak with a wholly abnormal voice quality (see further, p. 173). The ENT (ear, nose and throat) department of the hospital to which the patient was referred may not have been able to find anything physically wrong—no detectable pathology, in other words. Does it then make sense for this patient to be sent over to the speech clinic and immediately have his disability placed under the heading of 'speech (or language) pathology'? Thanks to an extension in the meaning of the term 'pathology' in the past 100 years, this should no longer be a problem. The word has been extended to the study not only of disease, but also of abnormal mental and moral conditions, since at least the 1840s, according to the Oxford English Dictionary. More recently, its sense of 'deviation from any assumed normal state' has become increasingly current, and the term 'speech pathology' falls within this development. Certainly in the USA, where there are more practitioners of this subject than in any other country, the designation 'speech pathologist' is the accepted norm. There is therefore plenty of precedent to use the term in this book's title—as long as the above limitations are borne in mind.

There is one other cautionary point to be made, before dropping the terminological theme, and that is to draw attention to another lexical nightmare, when it comes to labelling the subject-matter of study. We are proposing to study 'abnormal manifestations of language', it was said, cagily, on p. 1. Why not simply 'language disorders'? The trouble is that there are so many words, beginning mainly with 'd', which could be used to refer to abnormal language behaviour, but none of them mean exactly the same thing. They are all too restricting. They include: 'disorder', 'disability', 'disadvantage', 'disturbance', 'deprivation', 'disfunction', 'defect', 'distortion' . . . Certain of these terms have more radical implications of malfunction than others—'disorder', for instance, is plainly more deep-rooted a problem than 'disfunction'. Certain of these terms, also, relate specifically to a single academic or professional interpretation. 'Disadvantage' and 'deprivation' are more widely encountered in sociological and educational discussion of language problems. 'Disturbance' and 'disability' regularly have overtones of specifically psychological problems. 'Defect' reminds one of the days when a popular conception of a speech clinician was that of an 'oral engineer'—a curer of lisps and weak *r*'s. And so we could continue, trying to tease apart the associations of these various labels. It is probably not a fruitful line to take, in an introductory book; but it is important for the reader encountering this subject for the first time to realise that there is a problem here. In my view, the most neutral label is 'disability', and it is this which I shall generally use throughout this book. But the decision is, to say the least, somewhat arbitrary.

What counts as 'language pathology'?

When would you say that someone was linguistically 'disabled'— linguistically handicapped? Sometimes the disability is fairly obvious; but by no means is it always so. Let us begin with the most obvious case. Everyone would agree that if a person lacks ability in one or more of the main modes of communication (speaking, hearing, reading and writing), he is certainly going to be handicapped in life. And such disabilities are common. There are many who totally lack the ability to communicate in speech, or who are totally deaf, or who cannot read and write. But these disabilities, it should be noted, are not equal in importance. Of the four modes, the first two are fundamental. Assuming that a child grows up in a normal human environment,[5] speech will develop naturally—without formal training. Hearing, too, is a natural developmental capacity—a prerequisite for normal speech. By contrast, reading and writing do not develop naturally; they are more sophisticated skills, which have to be formally taught, over several years, and which many millions of people throughout the world have never learned.[6] And of the first two, it is speech which generally attracts the most attention, because it is so much more obvious a facility to develop than is hearing. Failure to cry or babble properly, in the first months of life, will usually be noticed and investigated; failure to hear, on the other hand, may not be spotted at all—and may indeed stay ignored until well into the second year of life, when the child's failure to respond to noises, or to develop early words and phrases, may make the possibility of deafness slowly dawn on the parents. It was of course this apparent dependence of speech upon hearing which led to the original labelling of people as 'deaf and dumb'—a label which these days is quite erroneous in its implications. With modern techniques of deaf education, it is common for deaf children to learn a great

[5] Sometimes this does not happen. There are many recorded instances of so-called 'wolf-children'— children who have been left to live (or die) in the wild—and these children learn at most a few animal noises. A two-part book which reviews the most well-attested cases is Lucien Malson and Jean Itard, *Wolf children and The wild boy of Aveyron* (London, NLB 1972). A film about Victor, the wild boy found in the forests of central France, was made by François Truffaut, *L'Enfant Sauvage*. But not only wolf-children are involved, as the tragic story of Genie illustrates. This child was discovered in 1970 in an American city at the age of 13½, having led a life of almost total deprivation and isolation. She was unable to talk and was severely retarded. The story of her attempted rehabilitation is told in Susan Curtiss, *Genie: a psycholinguistic study of a modern-day 'wild child'* (New York, Academic Press 1977).

[6] Even in Great Britain, there are around two million adults who are unable to read or write, or whose level of attainment is so low as to be unable to meet their needs, according to recent literacy estimates.

deal of speech; and conversely, there are types of disability where hearing is normal, but speech is absent or severely impaired (see Chapter 4).

Could there be anything more serious than the complete absence of ability to speak and hear? That there are indeed such possibilities becomes clear when we put the study of language into a broader context, of communication as a whole. At least if you are deaf and without speech, you can gesture and signal. But what if these aspects of communication are affected? It should be clear from this that while language is the main means of human communication, it is certainly not the only means. Communication can take place using *any* of our five senses (or six, if you include telepathy!). There is, firstly, the *vocal/auditory* mode, or channel, which subsumes the speech/hearing distinction already referred to. Secondly, there is the *visual* mode, whereby we can communicate by gesture, posture, facial expressions, and so on. Thirdly, there is the *tactile* mode, whereby we communicate by touch, as in hand-shaking, back-slapping, and other interesting ways. Fourthly, there is the *olfactory* mode— communication by smell—normally only important as a factor in determining our interpretation of our surroundings (as when a smell 'communicates' the impending arrival of a meal, or the presence of a chemical reaction or diseased tissue). Fifthly, there is the *gustatory* mode— again, not so important for our purposes, but plainly one of the means whereby we can gain information about the outside world (as when we deduce, using this sense, whether food has been well-prepared). The study of patterned human communication in all its modes is known as *semiotics*. Fig. 1 summarizes the main branches of semiotics, giving the technical

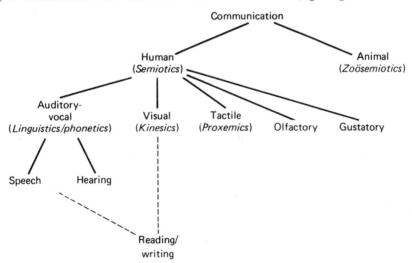

Fig. 1 The main branches of communication studies
Notes: (a) Animal communication has not been subclassified. (b) Note the overlapping status of reading and writing, dependent on both the vocal/auditory and the visual modes

terms sometimes used to identify the academic study of these areas.

Given this perspective, the possibility of more serious breakdowns in communication than in speech/hearing alone is perhaps now obvious. A combination of vocal/auditory and visual disability, for example, will pose especial problems. Such problems would identify the population of 'deaf-blind' children and adults—a term, incidentally, which includes anyone with a combined difficulty of hearing and vision, to any degree (in other words, the patient does not have to be totally deaf and totally blind). It is a disability which was first widely publicized when the story of Helen Keller was told. In such cases, we would have to develop a basis of tactile communication on which to work; and in fact it is quite possible to converse efficiently using a touch alphabet, where the various letters correlate with the position of one person's fingers against the other's hand. We can also extract a great deal of information by placing a spread hand against a person's mouth and neck, thereby picking up the various lip movements and vocal cord vibrations (see Chapter 3)—a kind of tactile equivalent of lip reading.

But what if the patient lacks even a tactile sense? With some severely mentally handicapped children, it is difficult to be sure whether even this channel of communication is open for anything except the grossest contacts. The child may be unable to do anything other than lie in certain positions, making minimal body movements. In such circumstances, the problem of communication is of course only one factor which has to be coped with, in ensuring the maximum wellbeing for the child. We keep trying to communicate, naturally, and to teach a communicative system of some sort, on the basis of whatever evidence we can detect of the child being able to control his behaviour; but progress is always extremely slow. Such cases, certainly, present language pathologists with some of their greatest problems.

Inability to communicate, at a fundamental level, presents a vivid picture, whenever it is encountered. But it has always been disability in speech, the primary index of language ability, which has attracted so much attention since the earliest times. One of the earliest references is in an Egyptian papyrus of around 3000 BC, which refers to the speechlessness that can come following head injuries. Many Greek and Roman scholars referred to speech problems. Aristotle, for example, in his *Problemata*, reflects: 'Why is it that of all animals, man alone is apt to become hesitating in speech?' Complete loss of speech, and stuttering: these are the two types of disability which are repeatedly referred to by writers of the classical and medieval world. The themes emerge strongly after the renaissance. Sir Francis Bacon, for example, wrote about stuttering (referred to as 'stut') in his *Natural history* (*Sylva Sylvarum*, 1627, Cent. IV, Sec. 386) (I have modernized the spelling):

The cause may be, in most, the refrigeration of the tongue, whereby it is less apt to move. And therefore we see that naturalls [i.e. idiots] do generally stut less, because it heateth; and so we see that they that stut, do stut more in the first offer to speak than in continuance; because the tongue is by motion somewhat heated. In some also it may be (though rarely) the dryness of the tongue, which likewise makes it less apt to move, as well as cold; for it is an affect that it comes to some wise and great men, as it did unto Moses. . . .

An interesting early account of the results of a stroke (see further, p. 86) was that of Dr Samuel Johnson. He suffered a stroke in June 1783, when he was 73, which robbed him of his speech, but left him able to write. From many letters describing his feelings, here is an extract of one written three days after the stroke:[7]

> On Monday the 16th I sat for my picture, and walked a considerable way with little inconvenience. In the afternoon and evening I felt myself light and easy, and began to plan schemes of life. Thus I went to bed, and in a short time waked and sat up as has long been my custom, when I felt a confusion and indistinctness in my head which lasted, I supposed about half a minute: I was alarmed and prayed God, that however he might afflict my body he would spare my understanding. This prayer, that I might try the integrity of my faculties I made in Latin verse. The lines were not very good, but I know them not to be very good. I made them easily, and concluded myself to be unimpaired in my faculties.
>
> Soon after I perceived that I had suffered a paralytick stroke, and that my Speech was taken from me. I had no pain and so little dejection in that dreadful state that I wondered at my own apathy, and considered that perhaps death itself when it should come, would excite less horrour than seems now to attend it.
>
> In order to rouse the vocal organs I took two drams. Wine has been celebrated for the production of eloquence; I put myself into violent motion, and, I think, repeated it. But all was vain; I then went to bed, and strange as it may seem, I think, slept. When I saw light, it was time to contrive what I should do. Though God stopped my speech he left my hand, I enjoyed a mercy which was not granted to my Dear Friend Laurence, who now perhaps overlooks me as I am writing and rejoices that I have what he wanted. My first note was necessarily to my servant, who came in talking, and could not immediately comprehend why he should read what I put into his hands.

Such an account might be compared with the more recent stories about the effects of strokes, illustrated below (p. 13).

Problems such as speechlessness and stuttering are obvious enough; but they by no means exhaust the range of topics which would have to be included under the heading of 'language pathology'. I shall discuss what this range consists of in Chapter 4, where each specific disability will be described in a separate section. Is it possible, in the meanwhile, to characterize language pathology in very general terms? Two such criteria have been suggested. First, language becomes a matter for concern when it impedes rather than facilitates communication. When it draws too much attention to itself, the listener or reader is distracted from the meaning which the speaker or writer is attempting to convey. Such a situation arises when

---

[7] Letter to Mrs. Thrale, 19 June 1783, No. 850 in the Chapman collection. It is reprinted in Macdonald Critchley's collected papers, *Aphasiology* (London, Edward Arnold 1970), 78.

speech becomes very weak or inaudible, or handwriting becomes too faint to read. It happens when speech, even though audible, is unintelligible, or when writing, even though visible, is illegible. It happens again when the speech or writing, although intelligible, is unpleasant—an abnormally harsh tone of voice, for instance, or erratic layout or line direction. If speech is nonfluent—full of hesitations and laboured pronunciation—there is cause for concern. Or when it makes use of sounds, grammar or vocabulary which are outside the normal range of the language to which the speaker belongs. The opposite of this is also a cause for concern: when a speaker *fails*, to some degree, to make use of the sounds, grammar or vocabulary of the language used around him, or uses these features in ways considered by the community to be inappropriate to his age, sex, occupation or the like. All of these factors will be encountered in our detailed discussion of types of language pathology in Chapter 4.

There is however one problem, against which the student of language pathology must always be on his guard. This is the danger of confusing a genuine difficulty of communication, for any of the above reasons, with an apparent difficulty, due to the prejudice or intolerance of the listener. It is often the case with regional accents, for example, that strong feelings are evoked: some accents are said to be 'nice' or 'musical', whereas others are said to be 'ugly' or 'harsh'. Most people have feelings of this kind, and their study is interesting in its own right.[8] The trouble comes when people attempt to impose their own standards of speech upon others, insisting, for instance, that a certain pronunciation is 'wrong' or 'slovenly', when in reality it may be the normal way of speaking for some social group. Such criticisms may take the form of a defence of imagined standards of excellence in a language—as one newspaper put it, 'Let us preserve the tongue that Shakespeare spoke!' At other times, these criticisms constitute a linguistic mask which hides an underlying distrust of the social values of the group involved. Either way, from the viewpoint of the language pathologist, such criticisms are beside the point. To attempt to change someone's accent or dialect when there is strictly no need to do so—or, putting this another way, when the only motivation to do so comes from an attitude of superiority— involves considerations of a quite different order from anything discussed in this book. In some ways, the different attitudes involved can be summarized by drawing a contrast between speech therapy and elocution. Elocution is the art of clear speaking in public, as judged by the cultural standards of the time; it aims to develop the speaking voice to its aesthetic and rhetorical peak, well beyond that which is necessary for the continuance of everyday communication. Unfortunately, as a profession elocution has often been associated with the instilling of attitudes of inferiority about one's natural accent or voice (as satirized, for example, in the figure of Henry Higgins and his attitude to Eliza Doolittle, in *Pygmalion/My Fair Lady*). When this

[8] See, for example, the review of the issues involved in P. Trudgill, *Accent, dialect and the school* (London, Edward Arnold 1975).

negative approach is absent, there is a lot that can be learned from the aims and insights of the elocutionist; but at all points, it should be plain, the concern of this profession is very different from that of speech pathology. A speech clinician is concerned to develop or restore language to an everyday norm, and would resist pressure to make this language conform to any real or imagined higher standards of aesthetic or rhetorical excellence.

So far I have talked generally about language pathology on the basis of factors which impede the communication of ideas using language. But there is a second criterion, much less obvious than the first, but often just as important. This refers to those cases where someone worries about his speech, without there being any real cause for him to do so. From the point of view of the listener, the speaker is communicating adequately—in terms of all the criteria mentioned above (audibility, intelligibility etc.). But the speaker nonetheless thinks that all is not well. He may feel his voice to be too high, or too harsh; may feel that his speech is unduly hesitant, or unpleasant, or inferior. This often happens after a person has undergone an operation which has altered the structure or function of his vocal tract: his 'new voice' may be much more efficient and pleasant than the old, to anyone who listens, but because he had got used to his 'old voice', the new voice may sound quite wrong in his ears. 'It's just not me,' one patient said, after removal of adenoids, which previously had made her speech sound quite indistinct. Such an attitude may not last long; but sometimes the upset caused by the change can take a great deal of sympathetic treatment to eradicate. And in other areas too, such as during the recovery of speech following a stroke, in stuttering therapy, or in certain kinds of psychological disturbance, such pessimistic attitudes are not uncommon—and are often quite deeply felt.

The effects of language disability

What is linguistic disability like? How does the patient feel? Such questions occur to anyone encountering this subject for the first time, and it makes sense to get as much insight as possible into the nature of these difficulties, at the very outset of our study. But where to get the information from? Unlike other forms of disability, the patient cannot tell us much, by definition! If he could, he would not be linguistically disabled. But in fact, it is possible to break out of this circle, to some degree, as the quotation from Dr Johnson will have shown. And there are now many books and articles written by the parents, relatives, friends and professional advisers of the linguistically disabled, as well as by the patients themselves, attempting to convey some insight into the nature of the various handicaps, and the acute effect they can have on family and social life. Take, for example, the opening lines of *The Siege*, by Clara Claiborne Park, which is subtitled 'The battle for communication with an autistic child' (Penguin 1972); here, the linguistic problem is only a part of a more deep-rooted disturbance, but its importance to the author is evident throughout the book:

> We start with an image—a tiny, golden child on hands and knees, circling round and round a spot on the floor in mysterious self-absorbed delight. She does not look up, though she is smiling and laughing; she does not call our attention to the mysterious object of her pleasure. She does not see us at all. She and the spot are all there is, and though she is eighteen months old, an age for touching, tasting, pointing, pushing, exploring, she is doing none of these. She does not walk, or crawl upstairs, or pull herself to her feet to reach for objects. She doesn't *want* any objects. Instead, she circles her spot. Or she sits, a long chain in her hand, snaking it up and down, up and down, watching it coil and uncoil, for twenty minutes, half an hour—until someone comes, moves her or feeds her or gives her another toy, or perhaps a book.
>
> We are a bookish family. She too likes books. Rapidly, expertly, decisively, she flips the pages, one by one by one. Bright pictures or text are the same to her; one could not say she doesn't see them, or that she does. Rapidly, with uninterrupted rhythm, the pages turn.
>
> One speaks to her, loudly or softly. There is no response. She is deaf, perhaps. That would explain a lot of things—her total inattention to simple commands and requests, which we thought stubbornness; the fact that as month follows month she speaks no more than a word or two, and these only once or twice a week; even, perhaps, her self-absorption. But we do not really think she is deaf. She turns, when you least expect it, at a sudden noise. The soft whirr as the water enters the washing machine, makes her wheel round. And there are the words. If she were deaf there would be no words. But out of nowhere they appear. And into nowhere they disappear; each new word displaces its predecessor. At any given time she has a word, not a vocabulary.   (9–10)

Here is another example, well into the story this time. It is an extract from Elizabeth Browning's story of her severely handicapped child, partially deaf and aphasic (a condition we discuss in Chapter 4): *I can't see what you're saying* (London, Elek, 1972).

> One day at tea-time Freddy was in his high chair when he suddenly saw something which reminded him of something else. The crying out began, and he had taken to making 'asking' noises. Jean said she had seen him with a match-box in the bathroom and rushed upstairs and returned with it, triumphant. She was met by a face with eyebrows raised in hope and a smile hovering. The ensuing disappointment resulted in a howl of rage and frustration and a hand and arm hit the matchbox away. Heather remembered something in the garden and rushed out for that but with the same result. We then all left the table and searched the house until, at last added to the pile of objects like so much Kim's Game, the cherished thing was found. By this time Freddy was banging his head on the high chair tray in agonies of frustration and crying and throwing himself about, and the rest of us were soon reduced to pieces of chewed string with our nerve-ends jangling and our patience extended to breaking-point. When the treasured object was finally found, the ensuing peace and calm was very alarming and much too un-nerving to be enjoyed. We all knew it would only last until the next time he lost something.   (18)

Stroke: a diary of recovery was written by Douglas Ritchie in 1960 (London, Faber & Faber). One year after the stroke, he felt like this:

> My speech? I might have had two or three stray words but I could not tell. In the Centre I rarely spoke to anyone. I had nothing to say and I was embarrassed because I could not say anything. I read all the spare time I had. In the ambulance, where I used to spend upwards of two hours daily with four and five people week after week and where I was less embarrassed, I used sometimes to try different words. One week I was optimistic and the next there was nothing. But I had no doubts about speaking as normally as I did before I had the stroke: it was a question of time and of finding the man or woman who could find me the switch.
>
> My writing was more depressing. I had only written 'Good luck, Clif' or a message like 'cigarretes' (spelt wrong—this might have roused my suspicions, but it did not), and for the rest made the excuse that I did not write with my left hand. But it was my mother's birthday in May and I felt that I should write her a letter. I no sooner had the paper in front of me when every single word galloped out of sight. I was left staring at the blank sheet. Nearly half an hour passed; panic grew; this was nothing to do with my left hand. At length my wife came in and she dictated slowly, letter by letter, 'many happy returns . . .'. I managed to forget my panic for a time.   (96–7)

These, and other accounts of the different types of disability,[9] testify to the all-encompassing, profound effect of language disability on all who become personally involved with it. The student commencing his studies of this field cannot fail to be affected by it. And yet, as with all the caring professions, he must learn to distance himself from it, otherwise his professional judgement and objectivity will be impaired. This is perhaps the central difficulty, as well as the attraction, of working in this field—whether as researcher or as professional: one needs to develop and combine the human qualities of mature and sympathetic caring with the academic skills of methodical analysis and interpretation. Both are needed for real insights into the nature of language disability. It is for this reason that this opening chapter has focused on both modes of knowing, juxtaposing ideas about terminology and theoretical frameworks, on the one hand, with personal anecdote and history on the other. It is a pattern which will recur throughout this book.

[9] For example, Valerie Eaton Griffiths, *A stroke in the family* (Harmondsworth, Penguin 1970); Virginia Axline, *Dibs: in search of self* (Harmondsworth, Penguin 1971); James Copeland, *For the love of Ann* (London, Arrow Books 1973); Paul West, *Words for a deaf daughter* (Harmondsworth, Penguin 1972; Susan Hampshire, *Susan's Story* (London, Sidgwick & Jackson 1981). See also J. Quicke, *Disability in children's fiction* (London, Croom Helm 1985).

2

Models of language disability

In the previous chapter, we have noted an extremely wide range of factors relevant for the study of language pathology. Where, then, should we begin? Before launching into a discussion of individual disabilities, it will be useful to try to get a general view of the field as a whole, and of the main scientific approaches to it. A normal procedure in scientific investigation, especially when we are dealing with a new or unformed field of study, is to attempt to impose some organization upon it, by constructing a 'model' of the field. The aim of the procedure is emphasized by the philosopher of science, Marshall Walker: 'the purpose of scientific thought is to postulate a conceptual model of nature from which the observable behavior of nature may be predicted accurately',[1] and a similar view is expressed by Stephen Toulmin: 'The heart of all major discoveries in the physical sciences is the discovery of novel methods of representation, and so of fresh techniques by which inferences can be drawn'.[2] Science, it has been said, is a continual search for fresh models; and language pathology is no exception.

Of course, this is not the everyday sense of the word 'model'. A clinician constructing a model of linguistic disability does not get out her plasticine and attempt to build a miniature copy of a brain or a palate! 'Model', in its scientific use, has a much more abstract sense—or rather, senses, for the study of scientific models has itself a long, interesting and controversial history, as any text on the philosophy of science will show. A model is part of the process of scientific explanation. It is a visual way of expressing an abstract set of relationships, such as have been propounded by some theory. It is a way of physically representing the complex ideas which constitute a theory, so that they can become more intelligible. For example, it is possible to discuss the principles governing the number and nature of the elementary particles of matter in abstract, mathematical terms; but most of us who have grasped a little of what has been discovered by this branch of physics have managed to do so by applying our minds to the models of the elementary particles, as presented in introductory texts and television programmes. Take, for example, the model of the atom, 'containing' a nucleus, which 'consists of' protons and neutrons, and is 'surrounded by' electrons; these in

[1] *The nature of scientific thought* (Englewood Cliffs, NJ, Prentice-Hall 1963), 5.
[2] *The philosophy of science* (London, Hutchinson 1953), 31.

turn are investigated to establish whether they may be 'built up' out of even smaller particles of matter (the elusive quarks and antiquarks). Because I understand what notions such as 'building' and 'surrounding' mean, I can begin to make sense of the claims of particle physics; without this, I should be lost. And the same applies to all areas of scientific inquiry, such as the models of molecular structure, or of geographical terrain (a map is a simple form of model), or of historical relationships (as in a tree-diagram of the kings and queens of England).

One thing all models have in common: they are simplifications of the reality they represent. Features of the reality are left out, and other features emphasized. The model would not be a model if it did not do this. The reason, of course, is that the purpose of the model is to help our understanding. If all a model did was simply reflect reality, containing all its detail, we would be no better off. If I look down on a battle scene, and ask you to explain to me what is happening, and you simply hand me a photograph of the battle scene, I am hardly helped! On the other hand, if you give me a diagram showing me the main dispositions of the troops, with each side coloured differently, and the movement lines marked by arrows, I am likely to be much illuminated. This diagram is a simplification, though. It omits innumerable details. There are no battle-scars or blood on my diagram. But the simplification was made for a purpose: the diagram tells me what I wanted to know, and therefore the omitted details do not bother me. All models are in principle like this one: their purpose is to illuminate an area of inquiry, and they are always designed for a specific purpose. Insofar as the features of reality which the model represents are the ones in which I am interested, the model will be helpful to me, and I will continue to use it. Insofar as the model gives me details which are not relevant to my aims, I will find it unhelpful. For instance, there are many possible ways of modelling the human body—representing its muscular structure, its nervous system, its skeletal structure, its blood circulation, and so on. If I am trying to understand the neurological basis of a speech disability, I will be much helped by the model of the nervous system, but hardly at all by the model of the digestive system.

Of course, this simple account only works if I know what I want of my models in advance. If I *know* my problem is a neurological one, then I can select my neurological model to help me organize my ideas. But what if I do not know in advance which model is most likely to help me? What if there are no models available at all to guide me in my research? How should I begin to model the functions of the internal structure of the brain, for example? or of social relationships within a community? In such cases, I have no alternative (apart from giving up!) but to attempt to construct a model for myself, using whatever analogies I can find from other areas of experience with which I am familiar. There will be a lot of guesswork, but I can check my guesses by observing whether the patterns I see in my model actually turn up in reality. Putting this more technically, my model will generate hypotheses about reality, which I can then subject to experimental test. Insofar as my model suggests fresh hypotheses to me—brand new ideas—I will be well satisfied. My model will be a 'fruitful' one. On the other hand, I must be cautious in using my model. The patterns I put into it may mislead me. They may make me think of reality in a fixed way, so that when I make my observations I end up seeing only what I want to see. This is a familiar danger. Scientist A says of B that B is 'blinkered', unable to examine his data in any way other than the one B originally devised. What A means by this, of course, is that he does not think B's model is illuminating, and that his own model is better. B, if we were to ask him, might think the same about A's model! To a considerable extent, science involves this process of comparison of the claims of different models, building on their strengths and attempting to avoid their weaknesses. If the weaknesses of a model become so great as continually to distort reality, in the view of the majority of scientists, then it will be dropped—though this process often takes many years, involving a great deal of heart-searching on the part of those involved, and sometimes involving harsh judgements from society as a whole (as in the case of Galileo).

Models, then, do four things: (a) they provide an intelligible representation of a theory; (b) they generate hypotheses for scientific testing; (c) they provide us with insights about our field of study; and (d) they tend to make us think along fixed lines. We cannot do without models, in our work, but we must always be critical of them, in case they lead us astray. This is why it makes sense to begin our discussion of language pathology by asking what models have been proposed to make sense of this field, and what their strengths and limitations are.

Where does language pathology get its models from? In fact, almost all the contributing disciplines have, at one time or another, suggested models for use in the investigation and treatment of linguistic disability. But it is possible to group most of the suggestions into two main categories. One category derives from the principles and practice of medical science, or its contributing disciplines (such as anatomy, neurology), and this is usually referred to as the 'medical model'. The other derives from the behavioural sciences (psychology and linguistics, in particular (see p. 40)) and is usually referred to as the 'behavioural model'. Both models have important insights to offer the language pathologist, and inevitably, as the above introduction will have suggested, both have their limitations. It is therefore essential for anyone interested in the study of language pathology to become well-versed in the aims and techniques of both of them, as a preliminary to investigating the characteristics of specific disabilities. In some cases, he will see the disability most clearly through medical eyes; in other cases, an analysis in behavioural terms will be more helpful. But in all cases, he is in the position of having to integrate the findings which the two models provide (see further, Chapter 3).

What are these two models? The medical model, as its name suggests, tries to classify and explain linguistic abnormality in the same way as it deals with any other category of bodily abnormality (i.e. disease). One of the chief features of this approach is the emphasis it gives to the identification of the cause, or causes of the disease. One treats the disease by attacking or preventing the cause. The behavioural model, by contrast, places no such reliance on the notion of cause, but begins with the description and analysis of the patient's abnormal linguistic behaviour in its own terms. The abnormality is compared with normal behaviour, and a treatment programme is drawn up which tries to relate the abnormal to the normal patterns, without reference to the original causative factors. The difference between the two models can be illustrated from their contrasting approaches to particular linguistic disorders—say, the kinds of speech problem following brain damage due to a stroke. The medical model would begin by providing information about the area of the brain that has been damaged, and the effects of this damage on the general wellbeing of the patient (whether there was any paralysis, for example). The patient's background would be investigated (his previous medical history, his home situation, and so on) and one would try to establish whether there was anything in the patient's life-style or other circumstances which might explain the occurrence of his stroke. One would try to establish correlations between these factors and the type of speech problem observed. Damage to the front part of the brain might produce a different kind of speech problem to damage to the back part of the brain, for instance (cf. Chapter 3). The main aim is to make a prediction (a 'prognosis') about the patient's future medical condition, and to decide what treatment, if any, to provide. Specific predictions about the kind and rate of linguistic recovery would not usually be made, in this approach, except in very broad terms.

The behavioural model would begin the other way round, by trying to describe in detail the characteristics of the patient's abnormal speech. The aim would be to see if there was any stability, or pattern, in the speech, or whether he had preferences for the use of one area of language rather than another. Any conclusions here would be used to form predictions about the patient's future linguistic behaviour, and about the way in which he is likely to respond to particular lines of treatment. The medical care of the patient, which would be being handled concurrently, would not be considered relevant, except insofar as it would dictate general restrictions on what it would be practicable for the patient to do. At no point does this approach have to concern itself with the patient's previous medical history, or with his damaged brain anatomy.

Of course, as soon as one paints the picture in this way, the artificiality of the exercise becomes apparent. The two models are not usually in conflict. Rather, they complement each other to a considerable extent, the first focusing on the patient's general condition, as a context for understanding his behavioural limitations, the second focusing on the patient's behaviour, within this medical context. The more the medical analyst can describe his patient's speech behaviour, the sooner will he be able to compare the relative efficacy of his medical decisions with different patients. Likewise, the more a behavioural analyst knows of the medical condition, the more he can make realistic recommendations for treatment, by working within the overall physiological limitations suggested by the medical study. The language pathologist needs to be able to interpret and draw from both models of analysis. Sometimes medical considerations will be predominant, in his work with the patient (after surgical intervention, for example); sometimes, he has no alternative but to work on behavioural lines (as in the many cases of linguistic disability where there is no known cause). Sometimes he has to resolve the conflicting recommendations about treatment which might come from the two models—as when the medical model might suggest the surgical removal of a growth in the vocal tract, whereas the behavioural model might suggest that the growth would go if an altered style of voice were adopted. While ultimately the medical wellbeing of the patient is in the hands of the doctor, the advice the language pathologist can provide about the patient's linguistic habits, and the linguistic demands placed upon him, will be of considerable relevance in ensuring that the correct decision about treatment is made.

Aspects of the medical model

Let us look in a little more detail at the medical model of investigation, which is the older and the more revered of the two. The language pathologist must be fully conversant with the central notions associated with this approach, if he is to cooperate with and interpret accurately his medical colleagues. To begin at the beginning. A person feels unwell and goes to the doctor. As soon as he arrives in the surgery, he becomes a *patient*.[3] The patient tells the doctor how he feels, thus providing the doctor with subjective evidence about the nature of his condition. Those aspects of disease which lead to complaints by the patient are known as his *symptoms*. The doctor takes a *medical history,* in which he attempts to extract from the patient everything that could have a direct or remote bearing on the presenting condition. There is then a *physical examination* of the patient, where the doctor aims to provide himself with objective evidence about the nature of the condition. Any physical manifestations of disease which he encounters are known as *signs*.[4] His main techniques here are well-known (though not always by their names)—visual *inspection* of the body, auditory investigation of the sounds produced by the various organs (*auscultation*), the use of his hands to feel the condition of the body (*palpation*), and the tapping of the body surface (*percussion*). Taken together, the 'signs and symptoms' of the disease enable the doctor to arrive at a judgement concerning the nature of the disease, either immediately, or after subsequent

[3] The psychological consequences of this change in social state are interestingly discussed by Jonathan Miller, *The body in question* (London, Cape 1978), esp. 49ff.

[4] In popular use, the term 'symptom' is often used loosely to refer to signs as well. The importance to the specialist of clearly distinguishing between subjective and objective evidence, however, is central.

investigations (such as blood tests). This judgement, and the process which led to it, is known as a *diagnosis*. To be more specific, the doctor makes a selection from a set of possible hypotheses about his patient's disease; by comparing one set of signs and symptoms with another, he aims to end up with one hypothesis which would explain most satisfactorily the present condition of his patient. A more precise name for this technique is *differential diagnosis*.

There are, actually, many 'kinds' of diagnosis, depending on the nature of the evidence the doctor uses in order to arrive at his final judgement, and several of these are used by the language pathologist in his specialised domain. In one account, by the American speech pathologist, Edward Mysak, there are listed eight diagnostic approaches of value to the speech and hearing clinician:[5]

1 We may begin with the process of *differential diagnosis* already referred to. In the context of language pathology, what we are doing is comparing the signs of linguistic disability shown in one patient with the various patterns of disability known to exist. For example, a child with poor pronunciation might have his mistakes analysed and compared with the kinds of mistakes typical of children who are deaf, mentally retarded, paralysed, and so on. This is a common procedure in language pathology, but of course its success depends entirely upon how much has been discovered about the patterns of disability with which the comparison is being made. It is also very dependent on accurate behavioural analyses.

2 *Clinical diagnosis* is based on the study of the signs and symptoms of a disability, without necessarily knowing about the factors which caused them. This too is a very common procedure in language pathology, where so many of the observed disabilities have an unclear or only a presumed relationship to an underlying cause. Most cases of stuttering, or of delayed language development in children, are diagnosed in this way. We may hazard a cause for the disability, but usually there are so many possible causes (e.g. brain damage, emotional factors, environmental factors) that this is a risky business.

3 *Direct diagnosis* is based on the actual observation of the physical abnormality presumed to be causing the linguistic disability, or of other physical signs that relate distinctively to the disability. In general medicine, one might have to use surgical techniques to establish the nature of the disease; in language pathology, more direct methods of observation usually suffice. For example, the strongly nasal, breathy speech of a young child may be directly diagnosed if he is shown to have difficulty moving his palate properly, using direct observation, or X-rays, or various devices for looking into the back parts of the mouth and throat. Relatively few linguistic

[5] E. D. Mysak, *Pathologies of speech systems* (Baltimore, Williams & Wilkins 1976), 69–75. In fact, he lists nine, but his ninth category, 'tentative diagnosis' (i.e. one based on available information, and subject to change) seems to me to be of a different order from the others. There is a time when most (if not all) diagnoses are tentative.

disabilities have a straightforward correlation with physical abnormality, however.

4 *Diagnosis by treatment* is based on the results of a specific programme of treatment: in the absence of clear signs and symptoms, and perhaps with only limited and unclear data to analyse, the language pathologist makes a guess about the probable cause of the disability, and commences treatment based upon this guess. If the treatment is successful, there is some support for his guess. For example, it may be felt that a child's language difficulty is due to an underlying difficulty in paying attention, but without any definite evidence that this is the case; if the clinician then proceeded to treat the child, with the aim of improving his abilities to pay attention, and his language then also improved, his diagnosis would have been confirmed—by treatment. Unfortunately, such clearcut cases rarely emerge: it is difficult to be sure that methods of treatment are focusing solely on the presumed cause of the problem, and not simultaneously treating some other aspect. To help the child with attention problems, for instance, the clinician will have to use language, to tell him what to do.

5 *Diagnosis by exclusion* is based on the elimination of all the possible causes which might explain a patient's disability, except for one. For example, a patient with a hoarse voice will be physically examined to see if it can be explained by abnormalities in his vocal tract; but once this and certain other physical possibilities have been excluded, one would have to conclude that the disability was psychological in origin (cf. Chapter 4). As with (2) above, however, it is always difficult to be sure that one has in fact excluded all the other possibilities, especially when the question arises of brain damage, about which so little is known.

6 *Instrumental diagnosis* is based on the use of clinical instrumentation, such as techniques for establishing hearing loss, or abnormal movement of the vocal cords, or brain scans to detect tumours (see further, p. 88). The pictures and measurements obtained are not of course an end in themselves; they still have to be interpreted by the clinician, and incorporated into his overall view of the patient. A 'laboratory diagnosis', based on the results of tests carried out on various tissues or fluids, is in the same position.

7 *Provocative diagnosis* is based on the results of inducing symptoms of a suspected disability in a patient. For example, to obtain a better sense of the extent of a patient's stutter, the clinician may alter his way of conversation to see if one style (e.g. asking many questions) produces more stuttering than another. Here, of course, he has to be careful to guard against artificiality: getting someone to do something in a clinic may be no real guide as to how they perform in the outside world.

8 Lastly, there is *group* or *team diagnosis,* based upon the combined approaches of a team of specialists, working in a single setting, such as a hospital. In a speech clinic, for example, we may encounter, in addition to a speech clinician, a range of people including an otolaryngologist, audiologist, pediatrician, neurologist, psychiatrist, social worker, plastic

surgeon and orthodontist, several of whose specialisms are discussed later in this book (see especially Ch. 3). Each specialist investigates the patient from his own point of view, using the diagnostic techniques referred to above, and their opinions are coordinated. In this way, a more complete picture of the patient's disability is built up than using any other means. Successful teamwork, however, requires a level of organisation and cooperation often unavailable in routine health service practice. The sending of reports about a patient from one agency to another is still the norm.

Diagnosis, then, in its medical use, is a decision made about the nature of a disease. Such distinctions as the above indicate the complexity of this concept in medical practice, and the need for care in using and interpreting the term. A similar complexity underlies the other major concept of the medical model, of particular importance to language pathology, the notion of *etiology* or (the older spelling) *aetiology*.[6] Etiology is the study of the causes of disease. It involves the study of both the direct causes of a disease (such as a particular virus), as well as of the predisposing factors which lead to the disease (i.e. those factors in the body or the environment which make the body susceptible to a disease, such as a particular skin condition, or a particular climate). It should be noted that etiology is *not* the term to use when describing the course of development of a disease in the body, once it has begun (the 'pathogenesis' of the disease) or the factors influencing its progress (the 'etiopathogenesis' of the disease).

There are many possible causes for disease, and a classification in terms of etiology is often encountered in medical texts—and the studies of language pathology. The main categories include:[7]

1 diseases of genetic origin, such as 'mongolism' (Downs' syndrome);[8]

2 congenital malformations (i.e. any structural defects in the body present at birth, such as a cleft palate (see p. 187));

3 injuries,[9] whether physical (wounds, burns etc.) or chemical (poisoning) (see p. 107);

4 diseases of biological (or 'biotic') origin, as caused by bacteria, viruses, fungi etc.;

[6] Most modern texts use *etiology*.

[7] The present classification is based on the exposition of 'Human disease' in the *Encyclopedia Britannica* article by S. L. Robbins and J. H. Robbins, Macropedia 5 847–63. Alternative systems are presented in A. D. Thomson and R. E. Cotton, *Lecture notes on pathology* (Oxford, Blackwell, 2nd edn, 1968), J. Macleod (ed.), *Davidson's principles and practice of medicine* (London, Churchill Livingstone, 11th edn, 1974).

[8] The term 'mongolism' is a popular but somewhat misleading label: there is only the most superficial of resemblances to children of Mongolian descent. The usual medical label for the group of physical and mental characteristics involved (broad flat face, eyes slanting upwards, enlarged tongue and lips, small nose, sloping chin; heart/kidney malformation; abnormal patterns on hands and feet; slow reflexes; mental retardation) is 'Downs' syndrome', after the English physician, J. L. H. Downs (1828–96).

[9] The medical term for an injury or wound to the body (as opposed to the gradual emergence of disease) is *trauma;* one might thus talk of 'traumatic' etiology here. This term has also a popular sense, however, with which it should not be confused, referring to the deep impression caused by an emotional shock—a sense which in fact derives from psychiatry.

5 diseases of abnormal cell growth, as with tumours (or *neoplasms*); alternatively, we may talk of diseases of 'neoplastic' origin (see p. 107);

6 diseases of metabolic origin (i.e. of abnormal internal chemical reactions, as with hormone disturbances (cf. p. 176));

7 diseases of nutritional origin, whether of excess or deficiency;

8 diseases of immune origin (i.e. a disturbance in the immunity system that normally protects against disease);

9 diseases of psychogenic origin—the various forms of mental disease (insofar as this is the best way of describing them; see p. 67);

10 diseases of senescence (i.e. which accompany the process of aging), such as hardening of the arteries ('arteriosclerosis') (c.f. p. 177).

In addition, we should add a category of diseases of unknown (or 'idiopathic') origin.

I should emphasize that this is only one way of grouping diseases in terms of their causes. Other systems of etiological classification exist, based on different interpretations of the available evidence (such as the relative weight to give to genetic v. environmental factors). Moreover, there are other ways of classifying disease than the etiological one. These too have had their influence in providing models for the study of linguistic disability. In particular, we should note the following:

(a) *topographical* classification, in which diseases are classified in terms of the bodily system they affect, e.g. chest disease, abdominal disease;

(b) *anatomical* classification, in which diseases are classified in terms of the specific organs or tissues affected, e.g. heart disease, lung disease;

(c) *physiological* classification, in which diseases are classified in terms of the functional disability produced, such as respiratory disease, or endocrine imbalance;[10]

(d) *pathological* classification, in which the nature of the disease process itself is the basis of the classification, e.g. tumorous and other growths.

There are other possible bases of classification, for example in terms of incidence (i.e. the rate at which new cases of a disease occur, see p. 194), or in terms of legal implications (should a disease require legislation to safeguard the community, for example). But the ones mentioned above are the most important for present purposes. Distinctions of this kind will be found to be directly applicable when we attempt to distinguish the various categories of language pathology.

While this account is in no way an adequate coverage of the main aims of medical science, it will I hope suffice to indicate the kind of orientation which comes to language pathology from this tradition. It is also important to note the relationship between the two subjects: language pathology is not

[10] The 'endocrine system' is that system of glands which secrete hormones directly into the bloodstream, in response to instructions from the brain. Examples are the thyroid and the pituitary glands. Hormone imbalance in these glands may cause major bodily (e.g. sexual) abnormalities, many of which have associated linguistic difficulties, such as abnormal voice qualities (see p. 176).

to be *identified* with the medical model; rather, it *makes use of* this model. The language pathologist applied its concepts, methods and findings as part of his own investigation into the nature and treatment of linguistic disability. And in the process, several of the basic concepts reviewed above have come to be extended beyond their originally medical sense (as we have already seen in the case of 'pathology' in Chapter 1). To illustrate this, let us look at the relationship between 'signs/symptoms', 'diagnosis' and 'etiology', as encountered first in medical science, and then as a possible model for language pathology. The traditional[11] medical use is as follows:

Medical signs and symptoms

$\updownarrow$ DIAGNOSIS

Disease

$\updownarrow$ ETIOLOGY

Causes (direct and predisposing)

The language pathologist's frame of reference, however, is broader, as shown in Fig. 2.

In order to interpret this diagram, let us follow the case of Peter, aged 3, who is saying little more than a few words and phrases. Peter is referred[12] by his family doctor to a local speech and hearing clinic. The speech therapist makes an initial assessment of Peter's speech—in other words, an analysis of his linguistic signs and symptoms.[13] She concludes that there is indeed an abnormal development of language, compared with other children of Peter's age and background. She uses various tests to try to pinpoint exactly which features of Peter's language are most affected. Her diagnosis is 'language delay' (see p. 126). But what is the etiology of this disability? Unless this is investigated, the question of the best line of treatment will remain unclear. In terms of the present model, there are two possibilities, reflected in the two sides of the diagram in Fig. 2. Either there will be a medical basis for the problem, or there will be no known medical basis.[14] It is usual to investigate

---

[11] These days, many doctors extend these terms in ways very similar to those described below, as they interpret their role in the broader context, which includes a consideration of the psychological, social and other factors affecting the wellbeing of the patient. The problem, of course, is that the specialist skills involved in handling these other areas do not usually constitute a major part of medical training. The issue is controversial, so I have restricted myself to a traditional view in the present book.

[12] The process whereby a person is sent from one (usually medical) specialist to another is known as 'referral'.

[13] In fact, the distinction between 'signs' and 'symptoms' is not particularly useful in this case. When communicative ability is poor or negligible, there will be few expressed symptoms, by definition. All the therapist can go on is whatever signs of the disability she can detect in the patient's behaviour (as discussed later in this chapter). By contrast, this distinction can be helpful in such cases as stuttering, where it is often possible to distinguish a person's worries about his hesitant, unrhythmical speech (his symptoms) from the actual analysis of his speech patterns and accompanying behaviour (his signs) (see p. 166).

[14] 'Known' is important. The disability may have an underlying physical origin, e.g. an anatomical abnormality deep within the structure of Peter's brain; but if this cannot be established with our present techniques, the need for an alternative line of investigation suggests itself.

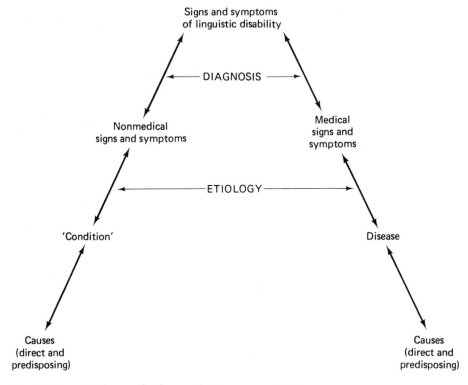

Fig. 2 Diagnostic frame of reference for language pathology

the medical possibilities first, as these are the factors about which most is known, and where guidelines for investigation are fairly standard. Peter is thus dealt with in terms of the right-hand side of Fig. 2. He has his hearing tested; he may be given a thorough physical examination; he may be seen by a neurologist. These investigations may indicate a clear medical cause, such as deafness. But what if everything is normal, in medical terms? There may be no physical signs which could explain the lack of speech, and there is nothing in Peter's medical history which might account for it. If there is no known physical cause for the disability, then the possibility of a nonphysical cause now comes to the fore (the left-hand side of Fig. 2). We have begun to diagnose by exclusion (cf. p. 20). It might be, for instance, that analysis of Peter's behaviour—his nonmedical signs and symptoms—shows him to be a very distractible, hyperactive child, who is unable to pay enough systematic attention to his linguistic environment to be able to learn from it. A psychologist's opinion would be essential here. Or perhaps Peter comes from a home background where he has been given little chance to learn from his environment—a social explanation for the problem. Or perhaps some combination of these circumstances is involved. In the diagram, I have put all these factors together under the heading of 'Condition', in an attempt to suggest that there is a comparable notion to that of 'disease' in the medical model, which can help to explain the linguistic disability. But it is only the beginning of the process of explanation. To say that his problem is 'caused' by poor social conditions at home is only the first step: what is the cause of the poor social conditions? What has to be treated first?

It should be plain from such a case study that the decision as to what constitutes the diagnosis and etiology of a linguistic disability is likely to be complex, and that the medical factors will be only one part of the overall explanation. Often, these factors may be the important ones; but rarely are they the only ones. Even if there is a clear medical condition demonstrated, it does not automatically follow that the cause of a linguistic disability will be solely medical. There is often a complex interaction between medical and nonmedical factors, which the language pathologist must do his best to take into account. The complexity is well illustrated by case histories such as the following, taken from Margaret Greene's study of voice disorders (see further, p. 173):[15]

Miss P. Aged 28 years. A grammar school teacher. She suffered from occasional loss of voice and catarrhal trouble but an X-ray of chest and sinuses showed them to be free from infection. Her voice was thin and high and lacking in resonance, and became hoarse after a day's teaching. Breathing was shallow and high and she was conspicuously tense and nervous. She had been troubled by catarrh for ten years and believed that her nasal passages had been traumatized at school when she had been shown how to blow through one nostril at a time. She sometimes coughed up blood and often woke choking at night. She lived with her mother who was separated from her father; she admitted to much home worry but did not wish to discuss it.

Instruction in relaxation and voice production was given and her voice improved steadily despite the fact that she never practised her exercises. Over a period of three months she gradually became more at ease and settled in mind and was remarkably grateful for the sympathy she found in the clinic and especially it seemed for the fact that although she was 'a psychological case' as she put it, she was never pressed for information. The catarrhal complex disappeared and a cold came and went without distress. She then asked to be discharged and on her last visit volunteered the fact that her father has been prosecuted by the police for some infringement of trade restrictions. She had felt acutely that his disgrace reflected on her and that her colleagues and pupils would think badly of her. Her acceptance with kindness and sympathy at the speech clinic had helped her to see her troubles in their right perspective, whereas prior to treatment her judgement had been altogether distorted by anxiety and the fear of ostracism.

The confession of her real problems came in this patient after the voice had become normal and speech therapy was no longer necessary. The positive attitude of the therapist and the exercises was the real healing agent. The unchanged

---

[15] Margaret C. L. Greene, *The voice and its disorders* (London, Pitman Medical, 2nd edn, 1964). Here and elsewhere in this book, I shall follow the convention of referring to adult patients by their initials—a practice which preserves their anonymity. The corresponding convention with children will be to refer to their first name, along with the initial of their surname, if needed.

attitude of the therapist after this 'confession' must have given her the final reassurance and security she needed.   (158–9)

Cases such as these, involving a complex mixture of medical and non-medical factors, are very common, and illustrate the difficulty the language pathologist faces in arriving at a clear diagnosis and establishing a definite etiology.

The medical model, then, is traditionally felt to be an essential part of any language pathologist's training, because it provides him with a standard procedure of investigation, and a body of knowledge which can be used as an initial frame of reference for analysing linguistic disability. He has to be thoroughly conversant with this frame of reference for the simple reason that in a large proportion of cases some medical condition *is* involved, and while he is professionally concerned only with the linguistic problems his patient has to face, he must see these in the context of the wellbeing of the person as a whole. When the linguistic disability is associated, in a fairly straightforward way, with disease, there is obviously a strong case for discussing the problem in medical terms. For example, there are several linguistic problems associated with brain damage (see Chapter 3), and from the earliest times these were introduced and discussed in a medical context. The linguistic difficulties were judged to be of a certain type on the basis of where in the brain the damage had occurred. But often the medical model provides only the beginnings of an explanation of a linguistic disability, and often no explanation at all. For those disabilities where it is unclear whether there has been any disease, or where the person seems well in all other respects, the applicability of the medical model is less easy. To take an elementary question, should such a person who seeks help be called a 'patient'? For example, if you suffer from a stammer, and are otherwise perfectly well, and you go to see a speech therapist, would you expect to be called a 'patient'? Some centres for the treatment of stammering avoid this term, talking instead of 'clients'—a label which in turn has been criticized because of its 'business' overtones!

There is also a serious limitation of the medical model, from the language pathologist's point of view, as regards treatment. The medical analysis gives an indication of the body's probable limitations in responding to treatment (part of the medical prognosis), but it does not give any positive guidelines as to how the treatment should be carried out. For example, if John has been diagnosed as deaf, the process of medical diagnosis will indicate the limitations on John's hearing, and the possibilities of recovery, and these facts will be important to the clinician who must collaborate in a remedial programme; but the medical information by itself does not tell the clinician or teacher what language to teach first, or how to move from one type of linguistic structure to another. Likewise, we may know which area of a person's brain has been damaged following a stroke, and having this knowledge may give us an idea as to how far the patient will respond, and how far we may expect treatment to be successful; but this knowledge does not necessarily tell us which linguistic structures to rebuild first. To obtain help on such matters, we need an alternative way of identifying linguistic disability, other than with reference to the medical or nonmedical causes which gave rise to them. Rather than classify linguistic disabilities in terms of etiology, therefore, we can try to classify them in terms of the patient's observable behaviour.

Aspects of the behavioural model

The medical model is in principle a familiar one. Several of its terms (such as 'symptom' and 'diagnose') have come into popular use. The other main model used in language pathology is by no means so familiar. It is a more recent development, deriving from the progress made in such twentieth-century subjects as psychology, sociology and linguistics. It is difficult to know what precisely to call this model of investigation. 'Behavioural' seems closest to what is involved. In a label such as the 'behavioural sciences', we are referring to those sciences which study the observable behaviour of men and animals—psychology, social anthropology and linguistics, for instance. It is this general sense which is intended, when I talk of the behavioural model in language pathology.

The main problem with this label is that it might trigger off the wrong associations in the mind of a reader who knows about certain important themes in psychology and psychiatry; so perhaps I should begin by commenting on what the label does *not* refer to. In particular, it does not refer to the specific school of thought in psychology (and also in philosophy) known as 'behaviourism'. This school, associated in America with the names of J. B. Watson, Clark Hull and B. F. Skinner, and in the Soviet Union with Ivan Pavlov, restricts the study of man and of animals to their observable patterns of behaviour, ignoring any mental processes which are not directly observable and measurable, e.g. such notions as consciousness and introspection. While the student of language pathology shares the behaviourist psychologist's concern to describe accurately the observed linguistic patterns in his patients, he does not restrict his study to these patterns; he frequently needs to refer to his patients' intuitions, or feelings, about his language, and the models of language analysis he will use often rely heavily on the notion of personal intuition (see further, p. 38).[16]

There is a (related) restricted sense of the term 'behaviour' in psychiatry, too, and here again the concerns of the present book should be distinguished. Behavioural principles were applied in psychiatry in the form of 'behaviour therapy', a set of procedures whereby patients learned to come to terms with the psychological problems. One such procedure is

[16] In relation to the topic of language, the classical statement of behaviourist method in psychology is B. F. Skinner's *Verbal behavior* (New York, Appleton-Century-Crofts 1957). Its main critic is Noam Chomsky, for example in *Language and mind* (New York, Harcourt, Brace & World 1968). A classical philosophical reference is Gilbert Ryle, *The concept of mind* (London, Hutchinson 1949).

'desensitization', in which a phobia (i.e. an irrational fear—of spiders, for instance) is treated by getting the patient to encounter the feared situation in a gradual and controlled manner, the aim being to counter his anxiety by increased relaxation. Another is 'aversion therapy', in which the opposite approach is used: here an unpleasant stimulus (such as an electric shock, or a slap) is linked with the abnormal behaviour, in order to eliminate it. 'Behaviour modification' is a third label which needs to be distinguished. Sometimes it is used as another name for 'behaviour therapy', but it also has a restricted sense, referring to one specific technique used in this approach— the technique of 'operant conditioning' (the patient is rewarded in proportion to the extent to which he modifies his abnormal behaviour, in the expectation that the reward will motivate his further progress).[17]

In the present book, the phrase 'behavioural model' refers to a particular emphasis in our investigation, and not to a school of thought. Moreover, as this book is about (abnormal) linguistic behaviour, my main source of information will come from linguistics, which is the name of the relevant science. We shall later be looking at what is involved in linguistics, as an academic discipline (see p. 40). For the moment, we need introduce only some of the more general points involved. Basically, the study of language pathology involves five interdependent stages:

1 the description of the linguistic behaviour of patients, and of the linguistic behaviour of the clinicians and others who interact with them;

2 the analysis of these descriptions, with a view to demonstrating the systematic nature of the disabilities involved;

3 the classification of patient behaviour, as part of the process of differential diagnosis;

4 the assessment of this behaviour, that is, plotting the kind and degree of abnormality, with reference to normal behaviour;

5 the formulation of hypotheses for the treatment of this behaviour, and evaluating the outcome of these hypotheses as treatment proceeds.

A noticeable feature of this way of looking at things is the large amount of preparatory work which has to go on before the process of treatment can actually begin (a point made by those critics of the term 'therapy' referred to in Chapter 1). Before you can treat a patient's linguistic disability (stage 5), you must first have reasoned out in advance what particular aspect of his problem will be the best place to start (e.g. an aspect of his grammar, or pronunciation, or vocabulary). In order to decide this, you need to have carried out a systematic assessment of his disability (stage 4). But how do you assess someone's language? At the very least, you need to be able to point out the way in which the abnormal features of his language differentiate him from normal language users, and from other types of patient (stage 3). This means, in turn, that you must have been able to

[17] See, for example, H. R. Beech, *Changing man's behaviour* (Harmondsworth, Penguin, 1969); for the psychiatric background, see p. 67.

identify some kind of pattern, or system, in his abnormal behaviour (stage 2). And it is obviously impossible to work out a system if you have not first described the object of study (stage 1). Moreover, the more comprehensive and systematic you can make this initial description of the patient's behaviour, the more reliable and full of insight your subsequent judgements are likely to be.

How easy is it to carry out this process of investigation? In fact, it turns out to be extraordinarily difficult, for a mixture of practical and theoretical reasons. Let us look, first of all, at the basic task of describing the patient's linguistic behaviour. Put yourself in the position of the clinician. The first thing you must do is obtain a sample of the patient's linguistic behaviour which is typical of him—a 'representative sample'. The patient has come to your clinic in the local hospital, perhaps for the first time, and meets you for the first time. How typical will his language be? How typical would *your* language be—faced with unfamiliar faces and surroundings? There is obviously a difficulty here, in that it is essential to develop a rapport with the patient before you can feel confident that the kind of language he uses to you is similar to that which he uses at home and with his friends. Indeed, in very problematic cases, it may even be that the patient chooses to use no language to you at all, to begin with. This is often the case with young children, who may take a long time to get used to you—several weeks, if you are seeing the child only once or twice a week, for a half-hour at a time. And even when he does begin to show an interest in communicating with you, it may take an even longer time before you feel sure that you have a clear sense of the strengths and limitations of his linguistic system. One therapist, after spending a great deal of time in an initial session trying to elicit simple one-word, 'naming' sentences from a child by showing him a picture book, and asking him to say what the objects were in the pictures, was somewhat startled to hear him outside in the waiting-room informing his big brother 'me can do them word in there'! He had shown no sign in her presence of any ability to use such a lengthy sentence, nor had his mother given any hint that he sometimes at home came out with such things.

But let us assume that you have solved this initial problem, and are faced with a patient whom you have come to know, and who is at ease in your clinic—or perhaps you are at ease in the patient's own home (i.e. you have made a 'domiciliary visit'). What are you going to talk about? Or, putting this another way, does it matter what you talk about? It does indeed. Some patients, for instance, find it particularly difficult to talk about certain areas of vocabulary (such as parts of the body, or colours). Others find it possible only to talk about what is going on in the room around them; they are unable to discuss 'absent' topics, such as what happened the day before, or what will be on television this evening. Some patients find it difficult or impossible to answer very general, 'open' questions, such as 'What's happening in the picture?', but are able to answer a question where certain alternatives have been presented clearly before them (e.g. 'Is the man running or jumping?'). It is not usual to think of your conversation with someone as being a 'task' for him to handle, but that is exactly what you are doing with linguistically disabled patients. And part of your clinical skill will be to make his task, of understanding your language, as easy as possible, by trying to get your language at exactly the right level so that he will understand and respond. It is not an easy level to find. If you do not simplify enough, your patient may get disheartened. If you simplify too much, he may think you are talking down to him. 'Why does everyone talk to me as if I were stupid?' one stroke patient once complained. 'Why does everyone talk to me as if I were deaf?' complained another, deaf, patient, with equal feeling!

But let us assume that you have sorted out this problem, and have decided what kind of conversation you want to elicit from your patient—whether a carefully pre-planned dialogue, a spontaneous chat, or whatever. How are you going to record your conversation? Remember that you want to analyse this recording later, so a great deal of thought must be given to technical and practical matters. Where are you going to put the tape recorder? Will the patient be upset if he sees it? Will he want to destroy it (usually only a problem with children)? And again: Where will you put the microphone? If you want to hear not only what the patient says, but also what *you* say, how are you going to position the microphone so that you pick up both voices well—and at the same time exclude as many background noises as possible, such as passing traffic, children in the room next door, and the like? While the recording is in progress, how will you make notes so that the events in the room, invisible to the audio tape, will be remembered afterwards? So often, one listens to a tape several hours later, and encounters a particularly puzzling piece of language—or an even more puzzling silence—and cannot recall what the patient was doing at the time. One way around this problem would of course be to video-record the conversation. This is sometimes done, but the expense of the equipment and poor recording facilities (e.g. poor lighting in the clinic room) prohibits its routine use. In the absence of such equipment, you have to be on your toes to ensure that you do not miss a significant facial expression or gesture, which might indicate that one of your questions has after all been understood.

But let us assume that you have solved the problem of keeping an accurate record of the conversation, and of the context in which it took place. Your patient has gone home, and you now have all the time in the world to listen again to the tape and analyse what is there. Unfortunately, this ideal world rarely exists. When one patient leaves, the next may be waiting outside. And others after him. A few years ago, the average caseload of a speech therapist in the United Kingdom was estimated as being about 100 patients.[18] If only a proportion of these are being seen every week, bearing in mind the need for the clinician to fit in her paperwork, discussion time and other administrative duties, it is obvious that one of the biggest problems you have

[18] According to the Quirk Report (1972), 7.24. By 'caseload' is meant the number of patients on the therapist's treatment and observation register at any one time.

to face is how to find the time to do what needs to be done. The Quirk Report summarized the difficulties for speech therapists at the time as follows: 'because of deficiencies in staffing and supporting services the best use is not made of their skills, preventive work is left undone, and some categories of patients are badly served; and behind the people known to need speech therapy at present, there are the potentially far greater numbers whose need has yet to be measured' (55). One solution, recommended by the Quirk Report, is of course to increase the number of speech therapists available to do the work—and such an increase has in fact taken place. But this Report did not really anticipate the amount of extra time that would have to be found to carry out the more modern kinds of behavioural analysis which were being proposed by the new methods of training—and as a result, despite the extra numbers, there are still pressing difficulties over time in the present-day service. It is a problem which many speech therapists solve by reorganizing their caseload so that, at least for the more problematic cases, they give themselves some opportunity to carry out the careful description of their patients' behaviour that is a prerequisite of systematic treatment. But for many others, either for lack of training or of opportunity, they must be satisfied with much less.

But let us assume that this problem has been solved, and that somehow time has been made available for you to analyse your patient's language. How will you set about doing this? The right technical equipment will facilitate matters, if this is available. When you consider the many tiny details which distinguish the various sounds of speech from each other, or the speed at which sentences are often spoken, with words being run together in various ways, it will be evident that making a description of what is on the tape will not be a straightforward matter. One device which helps is known as a 'tape-repeater'. This is a loop of tape attached to a tape recorder. When the appropriate switch is pressed, it repeats indefinitely the last five seconds or so of tape, thus allowing you an opportunity to hear a problem utterance over and over. Only by dint of such repeated listenings can you sometimes be sure that you have written down *exactly* what was being said—and in fact in no conversation is it ever possible to get everything right. The tape-repeater, at least, ensures that whatever *can* be transcribed, will be, with maximum saving of time. But in addition to such technical assistance, you will need to have had considerable training in the skills of transcribing and describing speech. Note, first of all, this distinction between 'transcription' and 'description'. A transcription is a precise notation of all the sounds used in speech. It is technically known as a 'phonetic transcription' (see p. 42), and it has to be able to cope with all the possible sounds that the human vocal apparatus can produce. It is obvious, therefore, that our everyday alphabet will not have sufficient letters in it to enable you to write down all these possibilities. Special symbols and accents have to be used, and the sounds they reflect have to be recognized, so that the whole of a patient's speech can be written down precisely and consistently.

This process can be illustrated by comparing the way in which two patients said the sentence: 'The three little kittens jumped into the basket'. Without knowing what the symbols mean, it will nonetheless be obvious that two very different types of pronunciation are involved, neither of which would it be possible to distinguish using the standard alphabet.

[ðə 'fri: 'lıkəl 'kıtənz 'ʤʌmp ınu: ðə bà:skıt]

[də 'fwi: 'lıkl kìtənz 'dʌmpt 'ıntʊ də 'bæskıt]

Each symbol, of course, is only a shorthand way of referring to the way a sound is made. If we were to write out in full everything we did with our vocal organs when we uttered the sound *b,* it would take up a great deal of space. The symbol [b] is simply a convenient way of summarizing all this information.[19]

A related kind of skill is needed when it comes to describing the other features of the language used by the patient—in particular, the way in which he builds up his words, phrases and sentences (what is usually known as his 'grammar').In grammar, too, you need to be able to notate the various patterns of construction that the patient uses, and sometimes quite a complex-looking apparatus for labelling sentences is involved. Learning to recognize parts of sentences as clauses, phrases, subjects, verbs and objects, and suchlike, is as much an aspect of linguistic description as is the phonetic description summarized in the notations above (see further, p. 42).

We have only begun the task of carrying out a description of our patient's linguistic behaviour (stage 1 on p. 28), but already it will be apparent that the operation is an exceedingly complex one, which requires considerable professional skill if it is to succeed. Obviously, too, we must know a great deal about the nature of language before we even begin—for otherwise, how should we know what to look out for, in making our description? It is not enough simply to observe a patient in order to describe his behaviour. In fact, observation without information is valueless. Imagine your reaction if I asked you to go into a room and 'observe' someone, and to report back in five minutes. You would be confused, because you would not know what it was that I wanted you to look out for. The way the person scratches his chin, or sniffs, may be a noticeable feature of his behaviour—but are such points the ones that need to be noted? Presumably I do not want a detailed account of *everything* the person is doing, so your problem will be to decide which particular points are the important, or salient ones, for my purpose. So what is my purpose? What do I want to know? If I provide you with some information about this in advance—perhaps give you a set of guidelines to follow while carrying out your observation—you will feel much happier. At least then you will know what you are supposed to be doing, and be able to

---

[19] Phonetic symbols are usually put in square brackets, to distinguish them from the letters used in the everyday alphabet, and also from certain other types of transcription used in linguistics; see further, p. 42.

concentrate your skill in doing it. What, then, do you need to know in advance about language, which will enable you to see a pattern in the linguistic behaviour of the patient?

Language

The first thing is to be clear about what is involved under the heading of language. What counts as language? We have already seen (Fig. 1, p. 7) that language is not to be identified with the notion of communication. There are many forms of communication, it seems, and only one of these is linguistic. Language, it appears from Fig. 1, is in the first instance auditory-vocal communication, i.e. speech; in the second instance, it is the encoding of speech in the visual or tactile medium (as with writing, and some forms of signing). This seems straightforward enough, but there are three theoretical problems which we must anticipate, in order to be able to work consistently within this definition.

1 This definition disallows our using the term 'language' to refer to aspects of communication other than speech/writing/signing.[20] In other words, such popular expressions as 'the language of gesture', 'the language of the face', and 'body language' are taken, on this view, to be metaphorical extensions of the term. They are not literally 'language', it is argued, because there are crucial qualitative differences between what goes on in speech/writing and what goes on in facial expressions/gestures, etc.[21] Two criteria have been proposed as critical. The first is to point to the major difference in *productivity* between spoken language and gestural communication. Productivity refers to the creative capacity of language users to produce and understand an indefinitely large number of words and sentences. Words in spoken language are continually being invented and dying out. Fresh combinations of words are continually being produced and understood. It is probable that most, perhaps all the sentences in this book are new sentences to you, i.e. sentences that you have not read or heard

[20] There are separate problems as to whether all forms of signing behaviour, as used by the deaf for example, are properly called 'language'. Some systems of deaf communication are largely language based, such as the Paget-Gorman Sign System (see further, p. 135); others are largely concept-based, such as the naturally evolved British Sign Language. It should be noted that the term 'language' is used generally, regardless of the nature of the signing behaviour involved. Whether the term is in fact appropriate to all such systems is at present unclear, as very little empirical analysis of signing behaviour has been carried out. For an initial account of this area, see I. Schlesinger and L. Namir (eds), *Sign language of the deaf: psychological, linguistic and sociological perspectives* (New York, Academic Press 1978).

[21] A similar, extended sense characterizes certain behavioural processes and activities studied by psychologists, sociologists and others. In relation to child learning, for example, we often encounter the phrase 'the language of play'. In relation to social anthropological studies of culture, we encounter 'the language of ritual'. Sometimes, other terms from linguistic analysis are used in such fields ('the grammar of dance', 'the syntax of sex'). Such phrases are often simply figures of speech coined to make a particular rhetorical effect; occasionally they are a serious attempt to use linguistic models in order to guide scientific investigation of a previously unstudied topic. But in either case, they are far removed from the strict sense of language found in the present book.

before; and yet, because you have learnt the rules of the English 'language', you are able to decode these fresh combinations and arrive at their meaning. By contrast, gestural communication lacks productivity. Gestures are not continually being invented and dying out. Fresh combinations of gestures are not continually being produced. There are in fact a very limited range of gestures you can make using your hands, posture, face and so on; and similarly, a very limited set of meanings that can be communicated in this way. The Third Webster International Dictionary contains over half a million words. A 'dictionary' of body language would find it difficult to accumulate more than several hundred contrasts.

The second main difference between spoken language and gestural communication is in their internal organizations, or structures. The former displays what has been called *duality of structure*; the latter does not. Duality of structure refers to the way language is organized in terms of two abstract levels. At one level, language can be seen as a sequence of units, or segments, which lack meaning. Segments such as *p*, *t*, *e* etc. do not have any meaning in themselves. However, when they are put together into certain sequences, and we look at the larger units so formed, then suddenly meaning is found: *pet*. At this second, higher level of analysis, language has meaning. It is this capacity, to produce meaningful units out of meaningless segments, which identifies a behaviour as being a language. By contrast, normal gestural communication lacks duality of structure. The minimal units of body 'language' are, to begin with, meaningful: the closing of one eye, the raising of one eyebrow, the clenching of a fist. . . . These seem to be the basic units of body 'language',[22] and once used they immediately communicate a meaning. Moreover, if a sequence of gestures is used—say, a wink followed by a shrug of the shoulders—there is a clear and direct relationship between the units in sequence and the units in isolation: the 'meaning' of the wink, and of the shrug, is preserved, which again suggests the lack of any real duality of structure.

What does this imply for the clinician? It does not of course mean that she need not be bothered with these nonlinguistic aspects of communication— 'nonverbal communication', as it is often called. On the contrary, her role is to understand the whole of her patient's communicative ability, and she will need to take into account these other factors in evaluating such matters as comprehension. If she asks her patient a question, and he replies with a nod, then this is a very relevant point for her to note. And working on body 'language' may be a useful first step in making contact with children who are showing little or no interest in conventional speech. But such activities are no substitute for language. If a patient restricts himself to his natural body 'language' there is very little meaning that he can unambiguously communicate. To develop his potential for communication, the clinician has

[22] It might be possible to break some of these units down into combinations of (meaningless) features, and thus to demonstrate a limited kind of duality of structure; but attempts to do this for normal gesture systems have not so far been very plausible.

to come to grips with language sooner or later; and when she does, the qualitative distinctions discussed above will require her to cope with a fresh teaching and learning situation. Because of the differences between language and other forms of communication, there is very little that she will be able to carry over from her knowledge of nonverbal communication into her work with language. The sounds, structures and vocabulary of spoken language (and the corresponding forms of writing) present her with a much more complex, multifaceted and long-term problem.

2 Given the emphasis in the above discussion on language as 'auditory-vocal communication', the next clarification which must be introduced concerns this notion: are all aspects of auditory-vocal communication to be included under the heading of language? The answer here is no. To begin with, we must exclude from the notion of language the range of physiological reflexes which may have auditory/vocal expression, such as coughs, sneezes and snorts. These features may 'communicate' in a sense (e.g. that we have a cold), but they are not linguistic features; they do not 'belong' to a specific language, but are rather the inevitable consequences of a biological state, cutting across language boundaries. There seems to be little sense in the idea of 'coughing in French'!

There is a less obvious consequence of biological influence on our auditory-vocal communication. Our biological constitution exercises its influence on our speech, not only when coughing and sneezing, but all the time. As soon as we speak, a sound emerges which is unique to the individual producing it.[23] Its vibrations reflect the size and shape of the vocal tract, the anatomy and physiology of which differs (sometimes minutely, sometimes grossly) between individuals. Each of us, as a result, has a distinctive *voice quality*—a permanently present 'background' feature of our speech, which enables people to recognize us and derive certain conclusions about us, e.g. how old we are, what sex we are, how healthy we are. Against this background, we learn to speak and to identify the speech of others. In a strict sense, therefore, voice quality is not part of language; rather, it is a permanent accompaniment of language. (The nearest equivalent, in written language, is our individual handwriting—but the analogy is by no means exact, as often handwriting styles are formally taught, and thus shared by many.) Once we have 'tuned in' to voice quality, we discount it: because it does not affect the meaning of what we say, it does not have to be listened to. Instead, we concentrate on listening to the sounds, words and structures which are in the 'foreground' of speech.

This point has been summarized by saying that voice quality is not a learned, culturally specific feature, as is language. But this may not be wholly

---

[23] At least, it seems to be unique. If it is, then it should be possible to produce 'voiceprints' of individuals, analogous to fingerprints, and these might be used in such fields as forensic science. Attempts have in fact been made to develop this notion, and evidence from tapes has sometimes been accepted as evidence in a court of law. But the matter is highly controversial, as to be valid the system must be safeguarded against the possibility of 'voice forgery' (as in mimicry) and the distorting influence of the recording and playback equipment.

true. It seems very likely that, as we grow up, so we learn to use the voice-quality characteristics of the various social groups with which we interact, and these merge, in a way that so far has been impossible to identify scientifically, with the biological features of the individual. A person may sound male, for example, but is this voice quality the result solely of his anatomy and physiology, or has he 'learned' to sound male, by unconsciously imitating the voices of other males in his culture? At first sight, this may seem an odd notion, but the more we compare the voice qualities of males from different cultures, the more community differences in voice quality emerge. Some cultures have male voices which are lower, or louder, than others. Even within a culture (say, in Britain) there are obvious differences between the 'community qualities' of males from various walks of life and various parts of the country. In some jobs, for instance, a gruff, low male voice is required; in others, a more 'feminine' voice would be expected. Distinguishing the biological from the learned characteristics of such voices will obviously be extremely difficult. And the same scientific problem arises in relation to all the other kinds of information 'carried' by voice quality—sex, age, occupation, social class, region. . . .

The theoretical implications of this issue are important. It means that often our awareness of voice quality will have an effect on the way in which we interpret someone's speech. If someone says, 'I like your coat', in a 'straight' male voice, the effect will be very different than if he says the same sentence in an effeminate voice! Depending on how well we know the speaker, we may be able to make our minds up as to what effect is intended—is that the way he normally speaks, or is he 'putting on' a special voice? But if we do not know the person well, or at all, we may be at a loss to know whether what has attracted our attention is in fact a voice-quality feature (i.e. one over which the speaker has no conscious control) or a linguistic feature (i.e. one which he has learned from the community and which he is deliberately introducing into the conversation to make a special effect). There is plainly an uncertain area between voice quality and language. It is often just not possible to say with certainty: 'that is a feature of English' as opposed to 'That is a feature of John Smith', or again, 'That is a feature of English' as opposed to 'That is a feature of French'. It is a difficulty, too, which the clinician often encounters, especially in the investigation of voice disorders (see p. 173), and generally in deciding whether the tone of voice adopted by a patient was intentional or not.

3 But linguistic idiosyncrasy is not solely a matter of voice quality. If an acoustic picture were made of several people saying a sound such as [a] or [t], there would be many differences between the several pronunciations. There would be differences of loudness, pitch height, length and timbre (see further, p. 106). Not all of these would be audible, but they would be there. However, these idiosyncrasies would not affect the nature of the communication between us. If I say my [t] sound with a stronger force than you, it will not affect your understanding of me, or me of you. Both of us will say *teetotal* in different ways, but we will discount these personal differences, and pay attention to what our two versions of the word have in common. Similarly, if I introduce a lot of hesitation noises into my speech (*er*, *erm* etc.), or pause frequently, then you will again discount these, in attempting to get at what I am saying. You may find the hesitations irritating, and your irritation may get in the way of your attention, but in principle they are irrelevant to my meaning. The basic meaning of a sentence does not change, if it is said in a hesitant, as opposed to an unhesitant way.[24] Likewise, if I start a sentence off, and then correct myself, you will pay attention to my correction, and not to the bit of sentence I began with.

How do these features of speech (and the analogous features of writing, e.g. variations in handwriting, or crossings-out) affect our definition of language? They affect it in this way: that they must be excluded from the definition. It is not enough to call everything that comes out of the mouth 'language', in the sense of 'a system for communicating meaning', for none of these features do actually communicate meaning (except in the sense of footnote 24). They could not, because they are idiosyncratic features; and a prerequisite of communication of any kind is that the parties involved share the *same* system, or means, of communicating. It would not be possible for me to communicate with you if I spoke in a personal language of my own invention. In order for us to communicate, we must agree to use a particular means—a particular code, or language. And that means agreeing to a particular set of rules which govern the way in which the code, or language, is to be used. If we agree to use two flags, in various positions around the body, to signal letters, as in semaphore, then I cannot suddenly in the middle of a message start using three flags. The message would become uninterpretable, because we would no longer share the same system. And it is the same with language, though here the rules are more extensive and more complex. Unless we follow the same set of rules, linguistic communication is impossible. And the hesitations, false starts, self-corrections, and other features I use in my speech from time to time are not part of language because they are not part of the single system of rules governing the communication of meaning that are used throughout the community.[25]

What, then, are these rules? Where are they to be found? The answer is: within us. As a result of the process of learning our mother-tongue, each of us has developed an internal sense of what the regular patterns of our language are. It has been a largely unconscious process—though sometimes it becomes an explicit one, as when in school we are taught to use certain

[24] I may of course read things into the hesitant sentence that would not otherwise be suggested, e.g. that your hesitance 'means' reluctance, or nervousness; but the meaning of the words and grammar does not change.

[25] This is not to say that there are no rules governing the occurrence of such features, but simply that these rules are not of a linguistic kind, i.e. involved with the structuring and communication of meaning. For instance, our use of hesitation may be explicable at a psychological or neurological level, and certainly there are several strong tendencies governing the places at which we hesitate in speech (see p. 66). But this says more about the way we are internally processing this sentence than about the meaning of the sentence. Both aspects are of interest to the clinician, of course.

constructions and avoid others. And it remains a largely unconscious ability. Without formal training, people do not have the ability to *define* the rules governing the ways utterances may be constructed in their language. And yet everyone *knows* these rules, for they are able to recognize acceptable utterances in their language, can correct unacceptable ones, and even pass judgements on their typicality or appropriateness. For example, here is a list of six nonsense words, three of which have been constructed according to the rules of English pronunciation, and three of which have not. It is not difficult to distinguish the two types:

> bov vbo vob ovb blov lbov

Working out *why* some of these sequences might turn up in English, and why some do not, is however not a simple task—especially when you consider the whole range of the pronunciation system. Similarly, we can look at a set of sentences and decide which are acceptable and which are not. Here are some cases:

> The cat sat on the mat.
> Cat the sat on mat the.
> On the mat sat the cat.
> Sat on the mat the cat.

The job of attempting to define explicitly the rules governing the construction of acceptable utterances in language is carried on as part of linguistics, and we shall have to look more closely at what is involved in carrying out this task in due course (see p. 41, ff.). For the present, it is important simply to note that to learn a language is to learn the abstract system of rules governing the way utterances are constructed, and it is our *knowledge* of these rules which constitutes the real measure of our language ability.[26]

We use our *intuitions* as evidence for the psychological reality of the rules we postulate for our language. For example, if in a grammar book you are told that there is an active voice and a passive voice for sentences in English, as illustrated by such sentences as *The cat bit the dog* and *The dog was bitten by the cat*, you might well ask, 'How do we know that this is so?' The answer is: if you reflect upon the meaning of these two sentences, your intuition tells you that they mean the same, and that moreover there are lots of other sentences linked just as these are (*The man saw the car* and *The car was seen by the man* etc.). If you feel that these sentences are closely linked, then this is one of the things that a grammar-book writer should tell the non-English-speaking world about—and he does so using the labels 'active' and 'passive'

---

[26] This distinction, between our unconscious knowledge of the language's rules and our actual use of these rules when we choose to speak or listen, has been formulated by Noam Chomsky as the distinction between *competence* and *performance*. See the exposition in J. Lyons, *Chomsky* (London, Fontana 1977). I have not in this discussion referred to the many cases where there is an uncertainty on the part of the speaker as to whether an utterance conforms to the rules or not, e.g. *The man what I saw was angry*. Discussion of such cases forms a great deal of the subject-matter of linguistics.

as ways of summarizing all the sentences that share the characteristics of each of the two types above. A grammar, in this way, is seen as a formulation of the agreed intuitions of the native speakers of a language. One reason which would lead you to conclude that a grammar book was unsatisfactory would be if the book told you that it was alright to say such sentences as *Cat mat the on sat the*. It is of course unlikely that any grammar of English would do such a thing; but there are many less ridiculous cases over which there has been considerable controversy, e.g. should a grammar 'prescribe' that you should use such constructions as *The man whom* I saw . . ., or refuse to allow you to end a sentence with a preposition?[27]

For the clinician, this distinction between rules and usage, and the fundamental role of intuition in finding out about language, is of central significance. She too needs to be able to distinguish what is idiosyncratic and casual from the underlying linguistic system in her patient. Her main concern is to ensure that the patient learns rules for the language as a whole, and is not satisfied with using single sentences. It may not be too difficult a matter to teach a patient to say *The cat sat on the mat* (e.g. the therapist might just get the patient to repeat the sentence, a word at a time); but what has the patient learned about the abstract structure of that sentence? Does he realize that there are three main parts to that sentence (*The cat/ sat/ on the mat*), and that he could replace each of these parts with corresponding parts, to produce an inexhaustible supply of such sentences—*the cat/dog/man/ . . . sat/walked/ran . . . on the mat/in the road . . .*? This is a much more difficult task for the therapist. Moreover, in coming to grips with it, she encounters the main methodological problem which permeates the whole field of language pathology, namely that she has usually no means of reliable access to the patient's intuitions about his language. Apart from a very few types of cases, there is no way in which the patient can inform the clinician, directly or indirectly, about the nature of his linguistic system. A 10-year-old who is slow in learning his language cannot usually tell his therapist which structures he feels most confident about, which he is uncertain to use, or whether he thinks that structure X and structure Y are related in meaning. A stroke patient cannot usually comment directly on the nature of the language he has lost. Nor do such patients respond so promptly and efficiently to the clinician's linguistic guidance that she can immediately deduce from their responses what the nature of their linguistic system is. In all such cases, the clinician is on her own: she has to work indirectly, by carefully eliciting and monitoring the patient's linguistic behaviour, and looking within this for the patterns of usage that might provide clues as to the nature of his underlying linguistic system.

Moreover, there is no way of knowing in advance whether the system she might find is going to be a reflection of the system present in the community to which the patient belongs. Sometimes it is evident that the patient is using

[27] For a discussion of prescriptivism, see F. R. Palmer, *Grammar* (Harmondsworth, Penguin, 2nd edn. 1984), Ch. 1.

a reduced version of the language heard around him. In many cases, however, the patient is 'doing his own thing': because of his disability, which has prevented him from learning or remembering the normal rules of the language, he has ended up inventing rules of his own. The job of the language pathologist is to work out what these rules are. But the trouble is, you have no idea in advance as to what kinds of rules they are likely to be. It is a bit like being given a jigsaw puzzle which could fit together in dozens of different ways, to produce several different pictures. The language you speak is one solution to the puzzle. The patient is in the process of putting his pieces together in a different way—and you have no picture to follow. Moreover (before this analogy dies completely!) you do not know whether any of the pieces are missing, in the version he is trying to construct. Meticulous analysis is the only way to obtain progress. You analyse a sample of the patient's language, and work out some of the possible systems he might be using. Next time you see him in the clinic, you can structure the situation to see whether you can communicate successfully with him, using these ideas—in other words, you are trying to talk to him 'in his terms', at a level and in a way where you will have made communication maximally easy for him. If your analysis was right, and you found his system out, then the test will come if the patient's communicative abilities improve. If there is no improvement, then either you were wrong, or some additional problem has intervened. Either way, it is back to the drawing-board: more meticulous analysis, more formulation of hypotheses, more testing. It is a long-term, laborious, and altogether engrossing exercise, for its challenge is rewarded by progress in both human and intellectual terms.

Models of language structure

From the above, it should be clear that describing the linguistic behaviour of a patient requires the clinician to make several decisions as to what counts as language.[28] But let us assume now that these decisions have been made, and that what we have before us is a sample of language ready for description and analysis. How should we organize our description of this linguistic material? Or (putting the question in the terms with which we opened this chapter) what linguistic model shall we use to organize our data and guide our investigation? A balanced and properly technical discussion of the kinds of model available would come from the field of linguistics. For present purposes, all I need to do is provide an outline of the main characteristics of a linguistic model which seems useful for clinical purposes, as a perspective for the detailed discussion of pathologies in Chapter 4.[29]

[28] For further discussion of the question of defining language, related to the above issues, see C. F. Hockett, *A course in modern linguistics* (New York, Macmillan 1958), Ch. 64; J. Lyons, *Chomsky* (London, Fontana 1977), Ch. 2.

[29] For a more detailed exposition of linguistic models, see Lyons, *Chomsky*, Chs. 5–7. For further reading on linguistics, see J. Lyons, *Language and linguistics* (Cambridge, CUP 1981), R. H. Robins, *General linguistics: an introductory survey* (London, Longman, 3rd edn. 1980).

In this model, an initial distinction is made between the notions of *language structure* and *language use*. Under the first heading is subsumed all the formal features of language, as directly observed in a spoken utterance (or its equivalent in writing). Most views of language classify these formal features into three main types, which for speech are usually referred to as *phonology, grammar* and *semantics*. These are said to be the three main 'levels' or 'components' of language. They may be studied in various orders: some linguistic theories begin with grammar, some with semantics or phonology. Basically, what is involved in each level is the following.

Phonology
At this level, we study the way the 'sound-system' of a language (or a group of languages) is organized. The human vocal apparatus can produce a very wide range of sounds, but only a relatively small number of these are used in a language to express meanings. The sounds do this through being organized into a system of contrasts, the various words of the language being distinguished from each other by substituting one type of sound for another. For instance, *pot* is distinguished from *got* by the contrast between /p/ and /g/ at the beginning of these words. How many contrastive units of this kind are there in English? The answer depends a little on how you analyse what you hear, and what dialect of English you are studying; but in one influential account of southern British English, there are 44.[30] I have listed these contrastive units, or *phonemes*, in Fig. 3, along with some examples, because it will be useful for illustrating disorders of phonology in Chapter 4. It should be noted that it is usual practice to transcribe phonemes in slant brackets (see further below). There are of course many variations in the contrasts listed in Fig. 3 which I have not referred to. For instance, when the contrast between /t/ and /d/ is made at the beginning of a word, it is generally more forceful than if it is made at the end of a word (cf. *tin/din* and *bit/bid*). Also, the above list gives information only about the way in which a word can be split up into a single sequence of phonemic units, or *segments*: *big* has three phonemic segments, for example, /b/+/i/+/g/. Also within phonology is the study of the way in which words (and of course phrases and sentences) can be said in different tones of voice, by varying the pitch, loudness, speed and timbre. These tones of voice cannot readily be analysed into segments, and they thus constitute a different field of phonology— *nonsegmental phonology* (as opposed to the *segmental phonology* illustrated in Fig. 3). Nonsegmental contrasts also need to be transcribed, and usually a system of accents or numbers is devised to indicate what is going on in the speech. For example, *yès*, with a grave accent, might be used to mark that the pitch of the voice is falling from high to low; *yés*, with an acute accent, might be used to mark a voice pitch rising from low to high. The contrast in meaning would be evident enough: *yés* is the tone you might use if you were

[30] See A. C. Gimson, *An introduction to the pronunciation of English* (London, Edward Arnold, 3rd edn, 1980).

/iː/	as in	*seat*	/t/	as in	*tin*
/ɪ/		*sit*	/d/		*din*
/e/		*set*	/k/		*cap*
/æ/		*sat*	/g/		*gap*
/ʌ/		*cut*	/tʃ/		*chop*
/ɑː/		*cart*	/ʤ/		*job*
/ɒ/		*cot*	/f/		*fat*
/ɔː/		*caught*	/v/		*vat*
/ʊ/		*put*	/θ/		*think*
/uː/		*shoe*	/ð/		*this*
/ɜː/		*bird*	/s/		*sin*
/ə/		*swimmer*	/z/		*zoo*
/eɪ/		*say*	/ʃ/		*shoe*
/aɪ/		*sigh*	/ʒ/		*vision*
/ɔɪ/		*boy*	/h/		*hat*
/əʊ/		*know*	/m/		*mat*
/aʊ/		*how*	/n/		*not*
/ɪə/		*here*	/ŋ/		*sing*
/ɛə/		*fair*	/l/		*live*
/ʊə/		*sure*	/r/		*road*
/p/		*pig*	/w/		*wet*
/b/		*big*	/j/		*yes*

Fig. 3 The phonemes of southern British English

puzzled; *yès* if you were giving a definite answer. There are, as we shall see, disorders of language which affect segmental phonology alone, nonsegmental phonology alone, or both together.

Phonology is the study of the pronunciation system of a language. It is therefore very reliant on the associated subject of *phonetics*, with which it is sometimes confused. But there is a crucial difference. Phonetics studies the characteristics of human sound-making, especially of those sounds used in speech, and provides methods for their description, classification and transcription. It studies sounds in three main ways. Firstly, it studies the way they are made by the vocal organs (this branch of the subject is known as 'articulatory phonetics'). Secondly, it studies the physical properties of speech sound, as transmitted between mouth and ear ('acoustic phonetics'). And thirdly, it studies the perceptual response to speech sounds, as mediated by ear and brain ('auditory phonetics'). It thus is grounded in the anatomy and physiology of the human being, and in the physics of sound waves, and can proceed regardless of the language or speaker. The methods of analysis used in phonetics are valid no matter what language the speaker happens to be using. The subject is sometimes called 'general phonetics', for this reason, and it is this which is the essential difference between this subject and phonology. Phonetics studies all human sounds, regardless of the language they happen to turn up in; phonology studies only the way in which a selection of these sounds are organized within a particular language. The distinction is reflected in transcription: phonetic transcription is identified by the use of square brackets; a phonological transcription, as we have seen, by slant brackets.

From the clinical point of view, the distinction between phonology and phonetics is an important one. It is possible to have disorders which affect only the phonological system of a person's speech, the phonetic abilities of that person remaining intact. In such a case, the patient would be able to make all the sounds required in English, but would have difficulties in organizing these sounds into a system for making contrasts in meaning (see further, p. 180). Conversely, it is possible to have disorders which are purely phonetic in origin, and where the phonological system remains unimpaired. For example, someone whose tongue was slightly paralysed would sound phonetically deviant, but he might nonetheless be able to use his tongue enough to be able to make all the contrasts he needs to in English. He could make all the contrasts listed in Fig. 3, for instance, but several of them would 'sound odd'. But probably the majority of 'pronunciation problems' in patients' speech result from a combination of both phonological and phonetic factors, and these prove the most difficult to analyse.[31]

Grammar
As we have seen, the phonemes of a language combine to produce higher-order units that have meaning. The most widely-used term to identify these larger units is *word*—a notion which is relatively easy to identify in the written language (it is the unit surrounded by spaces), and somewhat more difficult to identify in speech (where there are few equivalent pauses). One way of defining grammar is to say it is the subject which studies the internal structure of words, and the way in which words combine to form larger units, such as phrases, clauses, sentences and sentence sequences. The two parts of this definition are sometimes summarized under separate headings. The study of word structure is called *morphology*. The study of word sequence (or, putting this the other way round, sentence structure) is called *syntax*. Many books see the field of grammar as divided up in this way—into the subfields of morphology and syntax—but not all theories of grammar make such a clear division between the two. In fact, there are more different models of grammatical analysis than of any other aspect of linguistic structure, and accordingly it is often this field which poses the greatest problems for the clinician. She must appreciate the strengths and weaknesses of the grammatical model she proposes to use. A patient analysed using, say, the generative grammatical theory of Chomsky, will look very different from one analysed using the method of grammatical description proposed by the British linguist, Randolph Quirk, and his colleagues.[32] But of course it is the same patient.

It will be useful to outline a few of the grammatical distinctions which will

---

[31] For further reading on phonetics and phonology, see J. D. O'Connor, *Phonetics* (Harmondsworth, Penguin 1973), P. Roach, *English phonetics and phonology* (Cambridge, CUP 1983), R. Lass, *Phonology* (Cambridge, CUP 1984).

[32] For an introduction to generative grammar, see A. Radford, *Transformational grammar* (Cambridge, CUP 1988). For the latter approach, see R. Quirk and S. Greenbaum, *A university grammar of English* (London, Longman 1973). ·

be required later in this book, and for this I propose to use terms relatable to the Quirk model, as this is the approach which is the most widely used clinically in Britain. There are, however, major parallels between this approach and that used by several other linguists. Five basic notions are involved: sentence, clause, phrase, word, and morpheme. The relationship between these can be illustrated from a single sentence:

The cat bit the dog and the dog bit the cat.

This sentence would be said to contain two *clauses*, linked by a *connector*:

The cat bit the dog   and   the dog bit the cat

Each clause can then be analysed into a series of *elements* of structure, labelled Subject (S), Verb (V), Object (O), Complement, Adverbial. In the present sentence, the Subject-Verb-Object structure is used (twice):

The cat bit the dog   the dog bit the cat
  S   V   O   S   V   O

An element of clause structure may be just a single word (as in *bit*), or may constitute a *phrase*:

the cat   the dog   the dog   the cat

Phrases might become extremely complex:

The big fat ginger-haired cat bit *the dog from down the street*

Phrases may then be analysed into their constituent *words*, and the words, in turn, may be analysed into their component parts, if any, as in:

dis- abiliti -es

The various prefixes and suffixes, along with the roots of words, are referred to as *morphemes*; these constitute the minimal units of grammar.

From a clinical point of view, each of these notions has considerable relevance. It is possible to differentiate the grammatical ability of patients in terms of whether their problems are primarily located at the level of the word, the phrase, the clause, or the sentence. Within one of these levels, moreover, it is possible to determine patterns of preference, as when a patient consistently omits verbs from clause structure (thus producing such sentences as *daddy ball*, for 'daddy kicked the ball', or *daddy garden*, for 'daddy is in the garden'). Two emphases in particular identify this approach in contrast with the traditional ways of analysing grammar sometimes taught in school. Firstly, there is little attention paid to the *length* of a sentence; rather, all the effort is put into determining the *structure* of the sentence, and evaluating its complexity. Two sentences might be equally long, after all, but very different in terms of their internal complexity. Compare:

The man and the dog and the cat and the mouse are in the picture.
The man who has been standing in the corner has just bought a new car.

Both sentences are 15 words long, but the second is plainly more complex than the first. Secondly, the notion of 'parts of speech' is not so important in this approach. Often, people have been taught that there are a fixed number of parts of speech—noun, verb, adjective, preposition etc. The problem with this old notion is that it is impossible to work with it without knowing something about the structure of sentences. If I ask you, 'What part of speech is *round*?', it is not possible to provide an answer, without first putting the word into a sentence. Compare the following uses of *round*; it is:

a verb in *we must round the buoy*;
a preposition in *it's round the corner*;
an adjective in *I see a round table*;
a noun in *it's your round*;
an adverb in *he turned round.*

In other words, in order to decide what part of speech a word belongs to, you must look at the sentence structure in which it appears—and that is why the approach outlined above spends so much time on matters of sentence structure rather than parts of speech. Sentence structure is the logical place to start; the parts of speech (or 'word classes') are brought in in passing, as the analysis proceeds.[33]

Semantics
Semantics is the study of the way meaning is organized in language. From one point of view, it involves studying the various grammatical structures outlined above to establish the range of meanings they express. We have already seen that the sentence *the cat bit the dog* can be analysed grammatically as having three parts, which were labelled Subject-Verb-Object. But we could attempt to define the meaning that these parts convey, in which case we might conclude that the 'meaning' of the Subject in this sentence is 'the doer of the action', the 'meaning' of the Verb is 'the act itself', and the 'meaning' of the Object is 'the receiver of the action'. This would be the beginnings of a semantic analysis of grammatical structure. Likewise, we can take the notion of the *word*, and ask not 'how does it combine with other words?' but 'what does it mean?' This is a quite familiar notion, in fact, for we are all used to seeing the meanings of words listed—in dictionaries. But a dictionary is only a starting-point for a semantic analysis of vocabulary; its alphabetical organization is a convenience when we want to look things up, but it is an irrelevance when it comes to studying the ways words relate in meaning to each other. *Aunt* is at one end of the dictionary; *uncle* is at the other. But it is obvious that these words have a very close relationship in meaning, and any useful semantic analysis ought to be able to show this. There are indeed many types of meaning relationship between the words of a language—antonyms, such as *good* and *bad*; synonyms, such as *punctuality*

---

[33] For an introduction to grammatical analysis, see F. R. Palmer, *Grammar* (Harmondsworth, Penguin, 2nd edn. 1984). For the application of this model clinically, see D. Crystal, P. Fletcher and M. Garman, *The grammatical analysis of language disability* (London, Cole & Whurr, 2nd edn. 1988).

and *promptness*; hyponyms, such as *cat* and *animal*;[34] and so on. The main business of semantic analysis is to establish the structure of the vocabulary, or lexicon, of a language—a task which has been carried out for only small areas of vocabulary, so far.

But in a broader sense, there is far more involved in semantics than the study of the meaning of items of vocabulary and grammatical structures. The concept of 'meaning' is so wide-ranging. It can include the whole question of how meaning is expressed throughout a text—notions such as plot, subplot and character. It can include the question of what has *not* been said, as well as what has been said, as when one sentence presupposes another (e.g. if someone asks you, out of the blue, 'When did you stop eating radishes?', the question presupposes that there was a time when you ate radishes—even though no actual statement is made to that effect). Again, it can include the intention in the mind of the speaker, as when someone says 'I feel cold' when he *really* means 'I want you to shut the window'. And then there are such little-understood areas of meaning as the expression of the emotions using tone of voice (cf. p. 41), or the expression of 'social meaning'—as when one's language gives away one's class, or job (cf. p. 36).

Given that we are in the job of helping patients to express and understand linguistic meaning, it is perhaps ironic that semantics, the branch of linguistics which might most be of assistance, is the least-developed branch of that discipline. But is should not be surprising when we consider how intangible a notion 'meaning' is—and how much of it there is to subject to analysis. The points of contact between semantics and clinical linguistic analysis are pitifully few; but this will undoubtedly be a major growth area in the next decades.

We can summarize what has been said so far about the structure of language in the form of a diagram (Fig. 4):

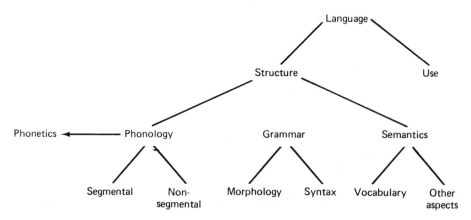

Fig. 4 The main branches of linguistic analysis

[34] Hyponymy expresses the relationship of inclusion—an X is a kind of Y. Thus, a cat is a kind of animal—but an animal is not a kind of cat.

Two supplementary points need to be made. Firstly, the model of structure can of course be extended to cope with the analysis of the written language. Writing has both a grammar and a semantics, so there is no need to modify the diagram in those respects; but instead of phonology it contains a writing system, i.e. a set of spelling and punctuation rules. The study of the writing systems of languages is known as *graphology*. Secondly, no further reference has been made in the above discussion to the study of language in use. Here we are referring to the ways in which the structure of language is made to vary, depending on the situations in which language comes to be used. For instance, when moving from a formal to an informal situation, from one job to another, or from one region to another, the kind of language used varies a great deal. Each utterance produced has nonetheless a phonology, a grammar and a semantics, of course; but the range of possibilities under each heading changes along with the situation. Thus a sentence such as 'what's up, me old mate?' has a different likelihood of occurrence, depending on whether the situation is a church or a pub. What is important, from a clinical point of view, is to be aware of the range of variation existing within the speech community, so that the patient's choice of language can be properly evaluated. Is the patient restricted to a single style of speech, or does he control a good range of styles? Do certain kinds of situation help him to use informal speech? What kind of language is the clinician using, in interacting with the patient? Is it a very different level of language from that which he is used to? Such questions raise daily matters of import, and need systematic attention. Much help here can be obtained from the relevant specialized branches of linguistics (sociolinguistics and psycholinguistics) and from the relevant areas of psychology and sociology, e.g. social psychology.[35]

Correlating medical and behavioural data

It should now be clear that the two models of investigation, the medical and the behavioural, provide very different kinds of information about a patient, and that both are necessary if we are to get anywhere near a full understanding of the patient's abilities and limitations, and a positive rationale for treatment and rehabilitation. One question remains to be answered: is there a one-to-one correlation between the findings of the medical model and those of the behavioural model? Does a given category of disease always produce the same kind of abnormal linguistic behaviour? If,

[35] Sociolinguistics studies the relationship between linguistic behaviour and the structure of society; (see P. Trudgill, *Sociolinguistics: an introduction* (Harmondsworth, Penguin, 2nd edn. 1983); psycholinguistics studies the relationship between linguistic behaviour and psychological processes (see H. H. Clark and E. V. Clark, *Psychology and language: an introduction to psycholinguistics* (New York, Harcourt, Brace, Jovanovich 1977)); social psychology is the study of human social behaviour (see R. Brown, *Social psychology* (London and New York, Free Press 1965), and below, p. 70). In the 1980's, much more attention has been paid to the interrelationship between language structure and language use, as part of the study of *pragmatics*: see G. N. Leech, *Principles of pragmatics* (London, Longman 1983) and below, Chapter 5.

for example, we brought together a matched group of children who had had a certain kind of cleft palate condition, or who were deaf to a certain degree, or who had a certain level of subnormal intelligence—to what extent would we be able to show the existence of 'linguistic syndromes'? Would all the deaf children speak in identical ways? Or the cleft palate children?

Perhaps running contrary to the expectations of the man in the street, the answer is no. No identity, certainly—and sometimes quite major differences emerge. The problem, of course, is the difficulty we have in matching the patients in the first place. Even if we match the group of cleft-palate children closely for age, sex, social class, severity of the cleft, and all the other factors which we know about, we are still left with several factors which we do *not* know about (see further, p. 191). Has there been any associated brain damage? How serious have been the ear, nose and throat infections the various children incurred? What kind of language has the parent been using to the children? Have the children been taught language in a more formal way? What about the varying emotional needs of the children? The questions could go on and on. What they amount to is an explanation as to why it is unlikely that there will be a very close correlation between a medically-defined group of patients and a behaviourally-defined group. And when the basis of the disorder is brain damage, as with mental retardation, or the aftermath of a stroke, then it becomes impossible to achieve any meaningful kind of correlation, in our present state of knowledge. One famous classification of the linguistic effects of adult brain damage (aphasia—see p. 140) illustrates this point well. Aphasic patients can be classified medically in terms of whether the part of the brain damaged is relatively forward or further back (the distinction between Broca's aphasia and Wernicke's aphasia—see p. 84). It is also possible to classify aphasic patients behaviourally, for instance in terms of whether their speech is relatively fluent or nonfluent. Some effort has been directed towards establishing whether there is a correlation between the two modes of description, and while there are indeed certain tendencies worth noting, there is plainly no necessary correlation. And the same conclusion is arrived at for any area of language pathology. As a result, so far, analysis of patients in medical terms has proceeded along largely separate lines from analyses in behavioural terms. The problems facing the speech therapist, who alone has to find a way of integrating the two areas in order to arrive at a self-consistent and systematic programme of individual therapy, are enormous. And for the language pathologist, interested in arriving at satisfactory conclusions about *groups* of patients, and thus developing a method of linguistic differential diagnosis, the problems are just as great. There are so many variables involved, both of a medical and a behavioural kind. In the next chapter, we will therefore look at one way of drawing the findings of these two models closer together, thus providing a possible basis for carrying out the kind of comprehensive investigation that needs to be done.

Other models

This chapter has made much of the major distinction between medical and behavioural approaches to the study of our subject; but it should not be forgotten that this way of looking at things is itself only a model of the field as a whole, and that there are other models that could be constructed in which either of these elements would be seen as less important, or in a different light. For instance, many behavioural workers would question the importance traditionally attributed to the medical model of investigation. We might avoid the medical/behavioural dichotomy altogether, in fact, by focusing on the contributing disciplines at a more specific level. If our interests were primarily in psychological disability, for example, we might model the field as in Figure 5a. As our interests are in linguistic disability, the field might be modelled as in Figure 5b. This model has much to commend it, because it places the focus of our attention, as language pathologists, firmly where it belongs; and it is in fact the model I prefer to use myself, when

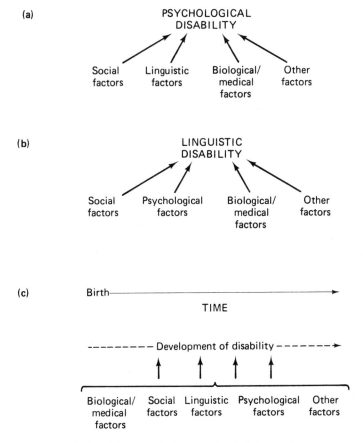

Fig. 5 Models of disability: (a) psychological emphasis (cf. p. 63);
(b) linguisitic emphasis; (c) developmental emphasis

engaged in research in this field.[36] But it would be premature to use it as a framework for an introductory book, as there are several theoretical problems which still need to be solved before the various components can be satisfactorily integrated, and there is a paucity of published studies which have so far used the approach.

A further limitation of the model presented in this chapter is that it views linguistic disability as a static phenomenon; the handicap is described 'synchronically' at a hypothetical point in time. A radically different model would conceive of disability 'diachronically', in terms of its chronological development, and might appear as in Figure 5c. A developmental perspective is an essential part of the study of linguistic disability, for two main reasons. It first provides a context within which we can specify what is 'normal' for a person at a given age, allowing for variation in social background, sex and other factors. Secondly, it helps us interpret the different effects of disability on the individual at different points in time. Whether the disability is *congenital* (see p. 21) or *acquired* subsequently, its natural progress can be plotted in relation to the individual's behaviour as a whole, and the effects of any clinical intervention monitored and measured, using the range of clinical assessment procedures which exist. This approach has come to be increasingly used in research and clinical practice in recent years, due to a coming together of interests from within medicine (*developmental pediatrics* or—the older spelling—*paediatrics*), psychology (*developmental psychology*) and linguistics (*child language acquisition*).[37]

It is pediatrics which has the most inclusive role, subsuming both medical and behavioural aspects of development. It is concerned to establish norms for all aspects of the physical and mental well-being of the child, in order to be able to assess variations from the normal, evaluate their handicapping effects on the child's health, education and social integration, and devise appropriate procedures of intervention. The pediatrician thus needs to be aware of the process of development found in the whole range of abnormal physical conditions (see pp. 21–2), and associated abnormalities in mental and social development (including language). Development is seen as a continuous process of change from conception, through birth to maturity, involving the simultaneous maturation of physical (especially motor),[38]

[36] See, for example, D. Crystal, *Clinical linguistics* (Vienna, Springer, 1981; London, Edward Arnold, 1987).

[37] For a general review, with particular attention given to the role of the contributing professions, see R. B. Johnston and P. R. Magrab (eds), *Developmental disorders: assessment, treatment, education* (Baltimore, University Park Press 1976) (though they restrict their title to handicaps arising out of abnormal brain structure, excluding abnormal physical development in general).

[38] 'Motor', as a neurological concept, is explained in Chapter 3 (p. 72). From a functional point of view, it refers to the body movements resulting from muscular activity. A distinction is generally made between *gross* motor skills, in which large muscle sets are used to promote locomotion, body orientation and balance, and *fine* motor skills, in which small muscle sets are used to promote specific, skilled activities, such as finger manipulation or speech.

psychological, social and linguistic skills. The way in which these different developmental processes interact (e.g. whether certain psychological developments necessarily precede certain motor or linguistic developments) is a prime focus of clinical interest, and an area to which the developmental psychologist can make a specific contribution.[39]

Developmental psychology analyses the changes in behaviour that take place with age, with the aim of establishing general principles governing the development of behaviour in children (and, sometimes, in adults). It avoids the physical, biological emphasis found in pediatrics, concentrating instead on the consequences of biological development for the child's mental growth and social integration. Important topics would include the differences in behaviour found in boys and girls (e.g. different rates of development of their various faculties, their attitudes to their gender roles in society); the role of the parent, siblings and peer-group[40] in fostering and interpreting the child's attitudes and behaviour, especially in the first years; and the development of individual differences (in intelligence, in particular). The work of the Swiss psychologist, Jean Piaget (1896–1980), stands out in its all-embracing coverage of the development of the child's mental (or 'cognitive', see p. 64) abilities. The behavioural effects of abnormality provide an important link with clinical studies, e.g. how the child compensates for sensory deficit, the effects of disadvantaged family or social background, or the consequences of nutritional deficits. Of especial significance is the extent to which there are 'critical periods' for the acquisition of specific patterns of behaviour, i.e. a biologically-determined timespan within the child's development, during which he will acquire a specific behaviour if environmental conditions are right.[41] It has been argued, in particular, that there is a critical period for spontaneous language acquisition in children, related to the development of the brain's physical structure (see Ch. 3), and that this period ends at puberty. Before puberty, it is maintained, children with brain damage affecting their language show remarkable abilities to recover spontaneously, whereas this is unlikely afterwards. The point is a controversial one, and very dependent on

---

[39] For further reading, see K. S. Holt, *Developmental paediatrics* (London, Butterworth 1977), R. S. Illingworth, *The development of the infant and young child* (London, Churchill Livingstone, 5th edn, 1972), J. O. Forfar and G. C. Arneil, *Textbook of paediatrics* (London, Churchill Livingstone 1973). For the development of the child *in utero*, see P. L. Williams, C. P. Wendell-Smith and S. Treadgold, *Basic human embryology* (London, Pitman Medical, 2nd edn, 1969).

[40] A peer-group is a group of people (in this case, children) who have a similar status in their own eyes and in the eyes of the society to which they belong. A child may belong to several peer-groups, e.g. in his neighbourhood, at church, in school.

[41] The notion of critical period is clearest in embryology, where if something interferes with the development of the embryo at a specific stage, subsequent growth may not make good the deficit, e.g. the failure of anatomical processes to unite in cleft palate children (see p. 188). The notion has also been applied to the development of behaviour in young animals, especially in relation to *imprinting*, the way certain species (of birds, in the original studies by the Austrian zoologist and pioneer ethologist, Konrad Lorenz (1903–)) form a rapid and permanent attachment to living things or objects, solely as a result of being in their presence. See K. Z. Lorenz, *King Solomon's ring* (London, Methuen 1952).

specialized studies of language acquisition to provide empirical data that bear on the issue.[42]

While psychologists have long been interested in language acquisition, particularly as it relates to the development of thinking and social skills, it is only in recent years that it has become a special subject of study in its own right. This has largely been due to the influence of linguistics, which in the late 1950s began to extend its concerns from a preoccupation with the adult language to include that of the child. Each of the main branches of linguistics (see pp. 40–7 above) came to be applied from a developmental point of view: thus we find 'developmental phonology' and 'developmental syntax' in particular, and the term 'developmental linguistics' sometimes used to characterize the field as a whole. The various branches shared the same aims: to establish empirically the order and rate at which the various sounds, words and structures in a language came to be acquired, and to develop a theoretical account of the observed processes of acquisition which would enable language development to be related to other psychological skills. Ultimately, it was hoped, universal principles, applicable to all languages, would be established and related to the general psychological principles which scholars such as Piaget were postulating. These aims are still upheld, but they are a long way from being achieved, due to the theoretical and methodological difficulties which have to be faced in doing child language research. Obtaining good samples of naturalistic data, setting up experiments in which all the relevant variables are controlled, interpreting accurately what the young child means in his early attempts to speak—these are but some of the methodological problems which hinder progress. Nonetheless, advances have been made, and the order and rate of emergence of several linguistic areas has been established with reasonable

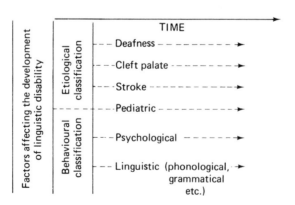

Fig. 6 Developmental factors in linguistic disability

[42] For further reading, see M. Donaldson, *Children's minds* (London, Fontana 1978), J. Nash, *Developmental psychology: a psycho-biological approach* (Englewood Cliffs, NJ, Prentice-Hall 1970), J. Sants and H. J. Butcher (eds), *Developmental psychology* (Harmondsworth, Penguin 1975).

confidence (at least for English and for some of the main European languages). It is this kind of information which will be referred to at various places later in this book.[43]

As we have seen, the developmental approach crosscuts the medical-behavioural classification used earlier in this chapter, and developed in the concept of the communication chain in Chapter 3. In order to incorporate it into my approach, it would therefore be necessary to introduce a developmental perspective into each disability, separately, as illustrated in Figure 6. In Chapter 4, therefore, when it proves useful to make such references, it is this general framework which will be used.

[43] For further reading, see P. A. de Villiers and J. G. de Villiers, *Early language* (London, Fontana/Open Books 1979) A. Cruttenden, *Language in infancy and childhood* (Manchester, Manchester University Press 1979), D. Crystal, *Child language, learning and linguistics* (London, Edward Arnold, 2nd edn. 1987), D. Crystal, *Listen to your child* (Harmondsworth, Penguin 1986), P. Fletcher & M. Garman (eds), *Language acquisition* (Cambridge, CUP, 2nd edn. 1986), P. Fletcher, *A child's learning of English* (Oxford, Blackwell, 1985), G. Wells, *The meaning makers: children learning language and using language to learn* (Sevenoaks, Hodder & Stoughton 1987).

3

The communication chain

One of the most convenient ways of drawing together the information provided by the medical and behavioural models of inquiry is to construct an even larger model in which the essential characteristics of both are incorporated. Naturally, such a model will be very abstract, and will leave out many details; but it is of value in that it can provide a sense of the relationships between the relevant variables, which would otherwise not readily emerge. This model is sometimes referred to as the 'communication chain', or the 'speech chain'. The latter is probably the more widespread use, reflecting the priority that most investigators give to speech over other modes of communication;[1] but it is important to recognize that the same model could be used for writing, signing or any other mode. Indeed, if we trace the history of ideas behind the use of this model, we will end up with the broadest possible view of the notion of communication, as developed within the field of *information theory*.

Information theory developed in the late 1940s, primarily as the result of proposals made by an American electrical engineer, Claude E. Shannon.[2] 'Information' does not here refer solely to its everyday general sense of 'factual knowledge', but has a much more precise interpretation. Under the heading of 'information' is included the whole range of signals that can be transmitted from one place to another, such as by radio or telephone, or within the circuits of electronic computers, or within the nervous systems of man and animals. The idea was to study the properties of these signals, and of the devices which send and receive them, to see if measures could be devised which would quantify the amount of information contained within a signal, the amount of information that a communication channel could transmit, and the capacity of a system to store and process information. The various practical applications of such studies are endless. An early application was in the field of telephone communication: how much speech sound could be omitted without the intelligibility or acceptability of the message being affected? could several conversations be transmitted at once

[1] The best reference is P. B. Denes and E. N. Pinson, *The speech chain: the physics and biology of spoken language* (New York, Anchor Books 1973).

[2] The classical textbook on the subject is C. E. Shannon and W. Weaver, *The mathematical theory of communication* (Urbana, University of Illinois Press 1949). An influential popular survey is C. Cherry, *On human communication* (New York, Science Editions 1961).

along the same channel? how much information could the channel cope with before it became overloaded? The analysis of the concepts involved required sophisticated statistical techniques, and the principles which came to be established were formulated in mathematical terms. The theoretical field involved is thus usually regarded as a branch of mathematics.

One result of this approach was an account of the information process in terms of a sequence, or chain of events—a chain which can be used as a basis for analysing what happens in *any* communicative activity. Basically, seven steps are involved. First, there must be an *information source,* which might be a human being, animal, machine, object (such as the sun, sending out radiation), and so on. This source has internal properties which enable it to construct a signal, or message: this process of construction is referred to as *encoding,* and this constitutes the second step in the chain. The third step is *production:* the encoded signal is made public—accessible to direct observation—through the use of some device (such as a nervous system, or a radio). The signal is then sent along a medium, or channel (such as the air, water, wires, nerves), and this constitutes the fourth step: *transmission.* Fifthly, the signal is *received* by some other device (such as a radio receiver, or another nervous system). The internal properties of the device which receives the signal enables it to be *decoded,* and this constitutes the sixth step in the chain. The remaining step is the decoded signal arriving at its *destination,* where the significance of the message will be registered in some way. We can summarize this process in a single line, as follows:

Information source→Encoding→Production→Transmission→

Reception→ Decoding→Destination

Sometimes the whole process is collapsed into three main stages:

Production→Transmission→Reception

and this in fact will be the usual use of these terms below. *Production* will refer to the whole process of making a linguistic message ready for transmission. *Reception* will refer to the whole process which takes place once a linguistic message has been transmitted.

This model can now be applied directly to the various stages involved in human communication. In some cases, however, it will prove useful to break down the steps in the process into 'substeps', in order to make the model more usable for the investigation of linguistic disability. Each step in the communication chain will require detailed study, but to begin with let us look at the process in outline, to provide a general perspective. A representation of the communication chain is given in Figure 7. For communication to take place, a minimum of two human beings are required, and these are symbolized by the facing heads. Communication may proceed in either direction. One person wishes to communicate a message to the other. The information source of the message constitutes step one of the process—the person's *brain.* The message is then encoded ready for transmission—but with a system as complex as the human being, in fact several substeps of encoding and transmission must be recognized. There is firstly *neurological* encoding and transmission: the message is encoded in signals capable of being sent through our nervous system. Then, at the end of this process, the neurological signals must be translated into *physiological* signals, controlling the movements of the relevant muscles involved in the communication process—those controlling the vocal organs, and hands and arms, in particular. This complex underlying system of physiological operations is, finally, manifested in the movement of the body structures used to transmit the message to the other human being—structures which need to be described *anatomically*. The analyst will have to pay particular attention to these last two steps—the anatomy and physiology of communication—as these are the most observable of all the processes in the chain. The language pathologist too will be primarily concerned with these steps, as they will be the first factors to check up on, in cases of abnormal development or use of language.

Everything so far has been concerned with communication from the point of view of *production*—how the message is produced in communicable form by the human being. The next step is the transmission stage *between* human beings. In the case of speech, the medium of transmission is usually air; vibrations produced by the movement of the vocal organs are translated into the molecular movement of air particles, which form sound waves—the *acoustic* step in the communication chain. In more complex communication situations, such as those involving telephone or radio, the sound waves are further encoded into electrical signals and transmitted using the devices

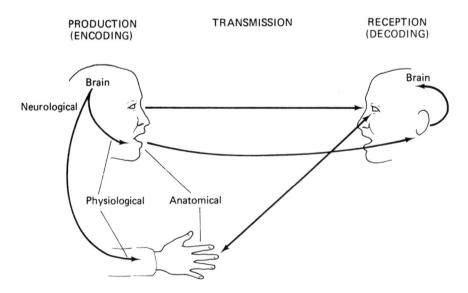

Fig. 7 The communication chain

available; but these aspects of the process are not really germane to the present volume. In the case of writing, visible marks have to be made on a surface of some kind—a *graphic* step in the chain. In the case of signing, configurations of hands, arms and face are set up and transmitted purely through the medium of light—a wholly visual step in the chain.

Whatever the medium of transmission, there comes a point where, if communication is to take place, the message has to be picked up by another human being: this is the *reception* side of the process, where the signals have to be perceived and decoded. Again, several substeps are involved. The *anatomical* step in the decoding process involves the ear and the eye (occasionally the hand). The *physiological* step involves the translation of these signals into mechanical movements underlying these receiving structures. These movements are in turn translated into nerve impulses—the *neurological* step in the decoding process—which ultimately reach the brain. This constitutes the destination of the signal, in the sense that it is here that the decoding process comes to an end, the signal's meaning at this point being interpreted. If all has gone well, the meaning which was in the mind of the first human being will have been effectively conveyed to the mind of the second. If it has not—if, that is, a wrong or misleading message has been conveyed, or no message at all—then the task facing the communications analyst is to find out why. Was the failure due to a breakdown in the communication chain at one or more points? If so, which? And what can be done about it? We are now plainly within the subject-matter of this book.

But before we proceed to look at these steps in communication in more detail, a few cautionary remarks are in order. The model in Fig. 7 may seem the 'obvious' way of investigating the communication process, but we must not forget that it is only a model, illuminating certain aspects of the reality and distorting others. For instance, there is really no clear dividing line between thinking of a message and neurologically encoding it, or between the physiological and the anatomical steps, or between production and transmission. How could an idea exist without the nervous system being involved in some way? How could we move a muscle without the relevant part of the anatomy being affected? How could we produce a signal without transmitting it? The reason why distinctions of this kind are made is that they simplify the task of discussing the problem—in our case, the problem of linguistic disability. I find the distinction between anatomy and physiology a valuable one, for instance, because I observe that some speech disorders seem to be the primary result of a physiological problem: the patient's anatomy seems perfectly normal, but he has difficulty in using it efficiently. And conversely, there are patients whose physiology seems perfectly normal, but who, because of some anatomical deficiency, are unable to communicate effectively. There are then many kinds of disorder where both anatomy and physiology are affected; but the fact that it is sometimes possible to talk about one without reference to the other is sufficient reason for separating them in the above model. And similar reasoning is involved behind all the other distinctions noted.

There is a further artificiality in Figure 7. The way I have explained it suggests that communication is a simple, linear, unidirectional process—A sends information to B and that is all there is to it. But far more is involved. The most important notion which has been omitted is *feedback,* another concept which stems originally from information theory, and which is of major importance in discussing several kinds of linguistic pathology. Feedback technically refers to the way in which a system allows its output to affect its input. A thermostat is a classic example of the way feedback operates: this device monitors the output of a heating system, turning the system off when it reaches a predetermined level, and turning it on again when it falls below a certain level. The amount of heat which the system puts out is 'fed back' as information into the system, and the system thereby 'told' whether it is functioning efficiently. In the present model, the system we are dealing with is the human being, and here too output affects input. The main means we have for doing this is the ear: while we speak, we are continually monitoring what we say. At a partly unconscious and partly conscious level, we are aware of what we are saying, and how we are saying it, and can compare this with what we intended to say. When there is a mismatch, we introduce corrections into our speech—correct any slips of the tongue, change the direction of the sentence (perhaps using such phrases as 'I mean to say', or 'what I mean is . . .'), and so on. These are examples of conscious self-correction. But at an unconscious level, feedback is continuously in operation, as can be demonstrated by interfering with the normal course of events. This can be done by delaying the time it takes for the sound of the speaker's own voice to be 'fed back' to his own ear. The process is called *delayed auditory feedback.* What happens is that the speaker's voice is stored for a fraction of a second on a recorder, and then played back to his ear through headphones, sufficiently loudly that it becomes the dominant sound to be heard. If the delay is of the order of one-fifth to one-tenth of a second, the effect is remarkable: the speaker begins to slur his voice and stutter in quite dramatic ways, and after a while may become so unconfident that he stops speaking altogether.[3] Evidently, the delay between the time it takes for the brain to initiate the right sequence of sounds and to interpret the responses has upset a very delicate balance of operation. The experiment demonstrates our reliance on feedback in normal everyday speech, and shows the importance of introducing a 'feedback loop' into our model of communication, as in Figure 8.

Auditory feedback is perhaps the most noticeable way in which we monitor our own communications, but it is not the only way. There is also *kinesthetic* feedback—the feelings of internal movement and position of our

[3] A similar effect may be produced if we try to talk in an extremely noisy environment, where we cannot 'hear ourselves speak'. The opposite effect can be produced, in the case of certain stutterers: using delayed auditory feedback, a temporary improvement to their stutter may be introduced (see p. 171).

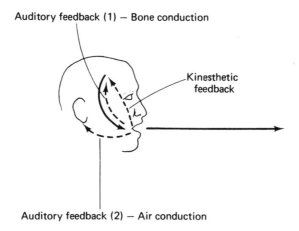

Auditory feedback (1) — Bone conduction

Kinesthetic feedback

Auditory feedback (2) — Air conduction

Fig. 8 Feedback in communication

muscles, joints etc. which we have while we are speaking, writing, or indeed performing any voluntary activity.[4] Knowing (at an unconscious level) where our tongues are in our mouths is an important factor in maintaining our clarity of speech. When this information is interfered with, as when we lose sensation following a dental injection, or obtain novel sensations from a new set of false teeth, our speech immediately becomes slurred. Likewise, our ability to write depends on a combination of kinesthetic and visual feedback. And lastly, there is a third way we have of obtaining information about our own voices, by monitoring our production of sounds through the bones and tissues of the skull. In fact, we 'hear' most of our own voice through this means, and not through the air to our ears: this is why we are usually surprised when we hear our voices on a tape recorder for the first time—we may not recognize ourselves, because we are used to hearing ourselves through our skulls.[5]

In recent years, the term 'feedback' has also come to be used in a looser, extended sense, which ought to be kept clearly distinct from the discussion so far. Here it refers to the way in which we monitor *other* people, as opposed to ourselves. It is plain that while we are talking to someone, we are constantly obtaining information from them as to how we are doing— whether our message is getting across, whether it is being misunderstood, objected to, and so on. The main means involved is our observation of the listener's face, but a very important factor is the way in which we tune in to how our listener verbally acknowledges the success of our message. Listen to a conversation, and you will notice that it does not consist of a sequence of monologues: person A speaks and then B and then A, and so on. While any

[4] The term 'proprioceptive feedback' is also used, referring to these sensations. The contrast here is with 'exteroreceptive', referring to impulses from sources outside of the body (such as pain, temperature), and with 'interoreceptive', referring to impulses arising within the organs and vessels of the body.

[5] For more on feedback, see D. B. Fry, *Homo loquens: man as a talking animal* (Cambridge, CUP 1977), Ch. 7.

one person is speaking, his speech is punctuated by an accompaniment of noise from his listener—a sequence of words which express such notions as agreement, 'I'm listening', 'carry on', and the like (*mhm, m, yes, sure, uh-uh* etc.). These become particularly crucial when one speaker cannot see the other (as in a telephone conversation, where to withold these noises will soon elicit an inquiry from the person speaking as to whether you are still there!). But they are an important feature of all conversational situations—and one, incidentally, which many categories of the linguistically disabled find difficulty in maintaining or acquiring.

A further limitation of the above model is that it says nothing about the *conditions* under which communication takes place—both the physical conditions (such as room size, environmental noise levels) and the social conditions (such as the formality of the situation, or the degree of rapport between the participants). As it stands, the communication chain has nothing to say about those types of communication problem which arise from circumstances outside of the neurological, physiological and anatomical state of the individual. If someone does not *want* to communicate, for instance, then this problem will have to be approached using other means. It may well be that, at some deep level of neurological reality, this attitude may be explicable; but in the absence of available techniques to demonstrate this, current assessment and remediation of such an attitude, when it is considered to be abnormal, will have to work with a quite different rationale. The importance of the above model in such contexts, of course, is that it provides a first step in investigation and diagnosis. It would not be right to conclude that the problem of non-communication was 'psychological' or 'social', in the *first* instance: rather, we should check that the various physical pathways for the communication of information were open—in particular, whether there was any deafness. Only then, after the range of physical tests had been exhausted, with negative results, would we move on to hypotheses of a psychological or 'functional' nature (see p. 68 and further, p. 123).

Lastly, an important limitation of the above model is that it does not tell us anything directly about *change* in the communicating system: it is a static model of communication, in the sense that it is a picture of what is happening in a communicative act at a given point in time.[6] Establishing that there is a breakdown at a certain point in the chain does not inform us of the etiology of the condition, nor does this model, as it stands, provide us with guidelines for remediation. Plainly, the model needs to be supplemented by whatever information can be obtained from both medical and behavioural standpoints, so that at each step a complete picture of the patient's disability is produced. Similarly, the model provides only a first

---

[6] In linguistics, the term 'synchronic' is used to label this perspective in relation to matters of language—where, for the purposes of analysis, language is studied regardless of its historical antecedents or current pressure for change. Synchronic is opposed to 'diachronic', referring to the study of language change over time—the historical study of language.

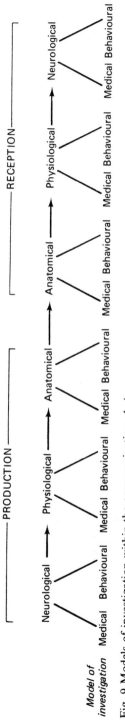

Fig. 9 Models of investigation within the communication chain

stage in investigating developmental disorders: for example, to illuminate the notion of 'language delay' (see p. 126), further medical and behavioural information is required. To show this, a fresh dimension needs to be incorporated into the communication chain, as shown in Figure 9.

For some disabilities, the medical contribution to the understanding of the breakdown process will be primary, and the behavioural will be secondary (for instance, a clear medical condition which resulted in predictable and unremarkable linguistic consequences, such as the escape of air through the nose which would follow from the failure of the palate to close off the nasal pathway (see p. 174)). For other disabilities, the reverse situation would obtain, as in the many pronunciation disorders in children, where there is no known etiology (see p. 180). Then again, in several disabilities, the contribution of medical and behavioural investigation can be mutually beneficial, the one informing the other, and it is here that some of the most interesting current research can be found (for example, in analysing the correlation between medical and behavioural improvement following brain damage).

The limitations of the communication chain model are several, but they are far outweighed in my view by its strengths. It enables us to recognize certain fundamental factors which will provide the basis for a classification of linguistic disorders (see Chapter 4), and suggests a way in which these factors might be related. It gives us an overview of a large part of our field of inquiry, and suggests a way in which our medical and behavioural modes of knowing might be integrated. It also makes us broaden our perspectives of analysis, by making us relate the findings of the different disciplines of study involved (anatomy, neurology, phonetics etc.), and thus helping us get to grips with the terminological, methodological and conceptual differences which separate these disciplines. But to be of maximum value, we need to know a great deal more about what goes on under each of the headings in the model. What actually is involved under the heading of 'neurological transmission' or the 'anatomy of the vocal organs'? In a short book, it is impossible to do anything other than provide an outline of the main issues, so that the examples of disability provided in Chapter 4 can be understood. Each of the sections which follow, it should be appreciated, would provide a major component of a course of study in language pathology.

Step 1   The brain

The brain may be studied from several points of view. An obvious approach is to describe its physical structure and mode of functioning in terms of neuroanatomy and neurophysiology, and this dimension of description will be introduced below (as Step 2). But in terms of the communication chain model, there is another dimension which must be seen as prior: here, the brain is seen as an 'information source', whose properties are analysed using the conceptual apparatus and methods of psychology. From the language pathologist's point of view, psychology plays a highly significant role, by investigating the whole range of factors which govern the brain's response to the outside world, and thus providing a framework of description within which linguistic issues can be related to other aspects of behaviour. When a language breakdown occurs, it may be possible to arrive at an explanation in solely linguistic terms; but more commonly, the explanation is largely or partly psychological, as when the deficit in the brain's processing ability turns out to affect other aspects of behaviour as well as language. From a clinical point of view, it will often be an important differential diagnosis, to determine whether a linguistic disability is a consequence of some broader problem (such as a difficulty in perception, or memory), or whether other psychological processes are normal. And an awareness of the main branches of psychology, and their clinical applicability, is consequently an important aspect of training.

Psychology is the scientific study of the behaviour of an organism (primarily, of man), and of the principles governing this behaviour as the organism interacts, socially and biologically, with its environment. For our purposes, we need look only at the study of human behaviour, ignoring the comparative aspects of the psychologist's work, in which the behaviour of man is related to that of other species.[7] Introductory textbooks on psychology classify its subject-matter in several different ways; but from the viewpoint of this book, one approach stands out as being particularly helpful, and that is to look at the psychologist's model of the brain as a series of processes governing the way in which we select information from our environment, organize it, and use it to construct our individual patterns of behaviour. Using the information theory model again, a threefold classification suggests itself:

> *input* processes—the way in which information is perceived, physiologically responded to and initially stored in the brain (see further, Steps 2 and 6);
> *mediating* processes—the way information, once received, is learned, organized and made available for future use (retrieved);
> *output* processes—the way in which this information is used to promote our biological and social behaviour, in relation to such notions as our motives, drives and skills.

The classification is convenient, though of course in several respects arbitrary. For example, it suggests that there is a basic division between the immediate storage of information (in *short-term memory*) and its more permanent storage (in *long-term memory*), whereas many psychologists believe a strong case can be made for seeing these two notions as being two different states of a single memory network. Each process subsumed under these general headings is, moreover, a complex field of study in itself.

---

[7] Study of animal behaviour is not entirely irrelevant; for example, studying the way in which chimpanzees learn to communicate using simple shapes has led to several interesting suggestions concerning teaching methods for the mentally handicapped. The chimpanzee study is reported in D. Premack, 'Language in chimpanzee?', *Science* **172**, (1971), 808–22.

Continuing with the example of memory, psychologists have developed several different experimental procedures, which have led to such distinctions being drawn as *recognition* memory (e.g. the subject learns one set of words, is subsequently shown another set and is asked whether he has seen any of them in the first set) and *recall* (e.g. the subject learns a set of words and is subsequently asked to say what they were). Then there is the question of how far our behaviour is facilitated when we engage in the process of *relearning*, and the process, difficult to study experimentally, of *redintegration* (the reconstruction of a past experience from a few clues, as when we remember an early event in our lives). The experimental verification of such distinctions constitutes a large part of academic psychology; and it is often possible to demonstrate their clinical relevance (e.g. an impaired ability to use recall memory but not recognition memory).[8]

This view of the brain, as an information-processing device, is a valuable one, for our purposes, as it permits the development of a behavioural framework for the study of psychological disability, in which each of the processes recognized is conceived as being theoretically independent from the others—thus producing disorders of attention, perception, memory and so on. These areas may then be subdivided, in terms of the sensory mode affected (e.g. auditory memory, visual perception, auditory attention) and several psychological tests have been developed in attempts to isolate and measure differential abilities in these areas.[9] The language pathologist will encounter several of these measures, as used in educational and clinical psychology, and they provide an important frame of reference within which specialised assessments and treatment procedures can be carried out.

Factors such as perception, memory and learning plainly constitute a large part of the brain's information-processing ability. Though each is a specialized area in its own right, they may be viewed collectively as an integrated set of processes involved in the brain's acquisition, organization and use of information—what is more succinctly referred to as *cognition,* and their study *cognitive psychology.* Under the heading of 'cognition' is included the whole range of factors involved in the notion of 'knowing', such as perceiving, remembering, paying attention, imagining, problem-solving, reasoning and evaluating. On this basis, we might postulate a cognitive 'step', as being the first movement along the communication chain, and this

[8] See further, P. Herriot, *Attributes of memory* (London, Methuen 1974), J. Greene, *Memory, thinking and language* (London, Methuen 1987)

[9] For example, the Illinois Test of Psycholinguistic Abilities (see Appendix) contains a series of 12 subtests which illustrates the application of several of these subdivisions: *auditory reception* (child produces yes/no responses to questions); *visual reception* (child finds a previously seen stimulus picture in one of four alternatives); *visual sequential memory* (child replicates a seen sequence of objects); *auditory association* (child completes a verbal analogy, e.g. *grass is green, sugar is —*); *auditory sequential memory* (child repeats increasingly longer sequences of digits); *visual association* (child points to one of four peripheral pictures most associated with a central picture); *visual closure* (child finds other objects like those seen in a sample picture); *verbal expression* (child makes verbal description of objects); *grammatic closure* (child completes a grammatical structure presented with ending omitted); *manual expression* (child demonstrates the use of pictured objects, e.g. hammer); *auditory closure* (child completes a word presented with sounds omitted); *sound blending* (child says successive sounds without a break).

is often done. But it is undoubtedly an oversimplification. It is by no means clear, in our present state of knowledge, how information is formed and stored by the brain, how many levels of storage there are, and at what point language must be recognized as a psychological reality. According to one view, we 'have an idea' which we wish to communicate, and this first of all exists in our brains independently of the language in which we wish to decide to communicate it. A second, separate step gives this idea a linguistic shape—an 'inner language', as it is sometimes called. According to another view, these two steps cannot be cleanly separated in this way. The act of thinking involves language, it is argued, and the formation of ideas in the brain presupposes their being given some kind of linguistic identity: there is no separate 'ideation'.

There is support for both views, depending on the kind of activity involved. Some types of emotional response, for example, plainly do not involve language: the feelings we have in listening to music, say, are not as a rule possible to 'put into words'. On the other hand, it is not usually possible to work out the stages through a problem (such as how to travel from place A to place B) without formulating the problem linguistically—and sometimes it proves essential to speak the problem aloud, or write it down, before our thinking can be clarified. When a child learns language, too, we can see both possibilities in operation; on the one hand there are many situations where the child obviously knows what to do with an object without being able to say what he is doing, to name the object, or to comprehend other people's language about it; on the other hand, there are many cases where the child seems able to organize his thinking only by having language available to do it for him (as when, for example, he uses colour-names to label the world around him). And, as a third illustration of the problem, there are evidently many cases of disability where, on the one hand, the patient has difficulty with thinking, *or* with language, but not both; and on the other hand, where the disability seems to involve both aspects together. Because of the many areas of difference, a distinction is generally made between 'cognitive organization' and 'linguistic organization', when we are discussing communication, the former being defined as above, the latter subsuming the range of structural and functional constraints modelled at the end of Chapter 2. The relationship between the two continues to be a major theme of contemporary research—especially within the interdisciplinary field known as psycholinguistics (cf. p. 47).

What this discussion amounts to is the view that there may be several 'deeper' levels of encoding going on within the brain, as communication takes place. Even within the 'level' of linguistic organization, there may be several levels of encoding. How, we might speculate, are the levels of phonology, grammar and semantics represented in the brain? Does the brain first of all 'generate' meanings, in the form of items of vocabulary, then put them into sentences, and then give them phonological shape? Or is a grammatical 'shape' first organized, into which vocabulary items are later placed? There are plainly many possibilities, and a great deal of research is ongoing into the extent to which there is evidence to support one or other of these models of language processing in the brain. For instance, it is evident that we do not plan our utterances 'a word at a time': if this were the case, our 'mental planning' would be reflected by the way we would hesitate and melodically shape our utterances. There would be a pause after every word—or at least, the same amount of pause after every word, with only the occasional variations due to changes in our attention, tiredness and so on. But speech is obviously not like that. We do pause, and shape our utterances melodically, but these features do not seem to relate to the way in which we use words, but to the way in which we use larger units of grammar. In particular, the clause (cf. p. 44) has emerged as a unit of speech which is more readily identified than any other as being phonologically 'shaped' by such features as pause and intonation (speech melody). We are much more likely to pause *between* clauses than *within* clauses, for instance. And if we do pause within a clause, then again it is not just a chance matter of where the pause will occur: the likelihood is that the pauses will occur between the main constituents of clause structure (between Subject and Verb, and Verb and Object, for example). Using this kind of information, it is then possible to draw conclusions about how the brain organizes the processing of speech.

Some interesting consequences follow. If it really is the case that the brain organizes and transmits information in the units which we call clauses, then it is very likely that if a mistake occurs in the organization process, its consequences will be most noticeable within the clause unit. Or, putting this another way, if something goes wrong within one clause unit, it is not likely to affect the other clause units in sequence with it. Some support for such a view has been obtained by analysing slips of the tongue. What seems to happen is that the vast majority of tongue-slips occur *within* clauses; they do not cross clause-boundaries. For instance, the following two examples illustrate, first, a likely tongue-slip, and secondly, a highly unlikely tongue-slip, happening to the (2-clause) sentence *John caught the ball, and Mary laughed:*

John *b*aught the *c*all, and Mary laughed
John *l*aught the ball, and Mary *b*aughed.

Tongue-slips are just one of the ways in which we can gain information about the way the brain works, with reference to language. But the evidence is by no means conclusive. Here, as in so many other areas reviewed in this book, there is a strong need for empirical research.[10]

Despite the theoretical difficulties of drawing a clear boundary-line between psychological and linguistic levels of organization within the brain, it is conventional to assume that a boundary-line *can* be drawn, and that

[10] For more on tongue-slips, see V. Fromkin (ed.), *Speech errors as linguistic evidence* (The Hague: Mouton 1973).

there are two academic modes of inquiry involved—one stemming from psychology and the other from linguistics. Either academic discipline can inform the other. For instance, a psychologist may use the linguist's ideas about language structure to help him determine how human memory operates, e.g. whether it is easier to remember certain kinds of information if it is previously organized into clauses of one type rather than another, or whether changing the intonational emphasis in a message will alter our ability to remember the message. By contrast, a linguist may use the psychologist's theories about memory in general to help him explain certain facts about the length or complexity of linguistic structures, e.g. why one type of structure might be acquired by children before another. A similar complementarity of approaches can be found in the study of psychological and linguistic disabilities. We can use the insights of psychology to improve our understanding of abnormal linguistic behaviour; and the insights of linguistics can be used to assist the study of abnormal psychological states. The relevant points of contact between these fields for the language pathologist are reviewed in Chapter 4 (p. 157 and p. 161). These points must however be seen in their full behavioural and medical context, where we need to be aware of several important professional and conceptual distinctions that are routinely made.

The main branch of psychology involved is known as *abnormal psychology* (or *psychopathology*): this is concerned with the scientific study of the abnormal behaviour and functioning of organisms, with particular reference to humans. Under the heading of psychopathology, the emphasis is on those disturbances which affect mental health, and the subject therefore includes—as well as the study of the theoretical relationships between such notions as mind, personality and environment—the analysis and evaluation of the therapies involved in treating abnormal conditions. The main branch of medicine involved is *psychiatry,* which is concerned with the diagnosis and treatment of mental disease—whether internal to the individual (his private thoughts and feelings) or external (his behaviour in the eyes of the outside world). The term *psychological medicine* is also used.

Mental illness covers a wide range of disturbances, ranging from mild emotional problems to the severest forms of mental abnormality. It is a highly complex and controversial field, containing several competing systems of classification and terminologies. One of the most traditional distinctions is that drawn between psychoneurosis and psychosis. Under the heading of *psychoneurosis* (or simply, *neurosis,* or *neurotic reaction*) is included a broad range of moods, fears, preoccupations and exaggerated traits about which a person is in some degree defensive or anxious. For example, a person may have an irrational fear of heights, or spiders, the fear being out of all proportion to the stimulus (what is known as a *phobia*). He may have an exaggerated concern over his health or bodily functions (*hypochondria*), or find himself acting in an obsessive or compulsive way (as in compulsive nail-biting, stealing, fire-lighting).[11] He may get abnormally depressed, or anxious, in varying degrees of severity, depending on the extent, duration and intensity of the reaction. And there are several other categories within the general heading of neurosis. *Hysterical* reactions are a further important subtype. Also known as *conversion* reactions, they refer to cases where aspects of a person's physiology fail to work normally, though there is nothing organically wrong. For example, mental stress of a particular kind might lead to sexual impotency, poor vision, or (cf. p. 178) loss of voice. What all these neuroses have in common is two things: the patient cannot readily control his reactions through his own efforts; and he is only minimally out of contact with reality—he generally recognizes the inappropriateness of his feelings and behaviour, and will often seek advice and help, especially from psychotherapy (see below).

In this respect, neurotic reactions are said to differ from the second main category of mental illness: *psychotic reactions, or psychoses.* These are major psychiatric disturbances, where the need for special, institutionalized control is usually apparent. They differ from neuroses in that here there is a fundamental disintegration of personality, with the patient no longer being aware of the abnormal nature of his condition, and accepting his behaviour as a normal way of living. A distinction is generally made into *organic* and *functional* types. Organic psychoses, as the name suggests, are disorders where there is a demonstrable physical abnormality in the brain. Examples include the major brain deterioration that may accompany aging, known as *senility* (*senile dementia*), the old person having little or no insight into his problems, and making no effort to care for himself. *Alcoholic psychosis,* due to excessive alcoholism, and producing delirium (so-called 'd t's'—*delirium tremens*) also has a physical basis. And there are several other brain disorders which affect normal psychological functions, such as epilepsy, arteriosclerosis, and general paralysis of the insane.[12] Functional psychoses, by contrast, are disorders where no underlying physical abnormality can be established (which is not, of course, to say that this does not exist—merely that none has been found, using present-day techniques). This is in fact a currently controversial issue in the main category of functional psychosis, *schizophrenia,* a disorder where there has been a disconnection of mental functions unintelligible to the observer. It is possible that a deficiency in certain enzymes in the brain may be responsible for the symptoms observed, in which case we should be dealing with an organic disturbance; but the point is disputed and so far unproven. Chief among these symptoms are major abnormalities and fluctuations in mood, unexpected (inappropriate,

[11] There is a distinction between obsession and compulsion: the former is a persistent *subjective* reaction, an emotionally-powerful idea recurring in a person's consciousness; the latter refers to cases where an obsession develops into an inner drive or impulse to do or say something—in other words, the reaction becomes *objective*.

[12] Insanity is often used loosely as a pejorative word; but in legal medicine it refers only to those suffering from a mental disorder of such severity that they are unable to manage their own affairs or are dangerous to themselves or to others.

dramatic) reactions to normal situations, social withdrawal, delusions and hallucinations. Schizophrenic states range from mild to severe (the latter including *catatonic* states, which often involve speechlessness, and *paranoid* states, in which the patient's deluded thinking has developed into a completely logical (to him) system—not only might he believe himself to be prime minister, for instance, but his entire way of life and modes of thought reflect this belief).

The psychosis/neurosis distinction is not always a clear one, there often being cases where the severity of the condition is apparently midway between the criteria referred to above. Similarly, there is often some indecision concerning the boundary-lines between these categories and the other forms of mental illness: *affective* (or *emotional*) psychoses, such as the various kinds of depression; *psychosomatic* disturbances (physical disorders apparently caused by mental states, as when anxiety is said to 'cause' ulcers or headaches), *behavioural* or *personality* problems (as in various types of addiction, or sexual deviations), and *mental retardation* (referring to those whose cognitive, emotional or social skills place them significantly below the level of the rest of their age-group). The field of mental retardation is of particular importance for the language pathologist, as so many of the children he will encounter will be mentally retarded to some degree (see p. 159), and he may regularly need to refer to the child psychiatrist, in order to obtain a full understanding of a child's capabilities and personality.

Child psychiatry is but one of the many specialisms which have grown up within psychiatry. Another is *psychiatric social work*, which deals with problems of mental health insofar as these arise from social conditions of home, work, environment and so on. But cutting across these professional specialisms is another division, in terms of the kinds of approaches advocated to provide solutions or progress in mental disease. There are, broadly speaking, two approaches to the problem. The first concerns itself essentially with biological approaches to treatment (*somatotherapy*), attempting to restore a normal bodily state through the use of medical aids. A major field here is the use of drugs (*chemotherapy*), such as tranquillizers, antidepressants, stimulating agents and so on. Alternatively, there is the use of neurophysiological techniques, such as the passing of electrical currents through part of the brain (*electroshock* or *electroconvulsive therapy*). In extreme cases, there is the possibility of *neurosurgery* to reduce excessively aggressive behaviour (a technique known as *pre-frontal lobotomy*, or *leucotomy*).[13]

The second main approach to psychological treatment is known as *psychotherapy*, sometimes referred to as the 'talking cure', in which patients have lengthy and regular interviews with their psychiatrist, with the aim of expressing, and thereby recognizing and controlling, their unconscious fears and problems. The term subsumes a wide range of techniques, such as those

[13] So called because it is the white matter tracts between the frontal lobes of the brain and the thalamus that are disconnected; see further, p. 80.

involved in psychological counselling, group therapy (as in Encounter groups) and the acting out of roles (in psychodrama), but above all it refers to the theory and practice of *psychoanalysis*, as propounded by the Austrian Sigmund Freud (1856–1939) and others (such as the Swiss psychologist, Carl Gustav Jung (1875–1961)). Psychoanalysis involves the minute analysis of the behaviour of the individual, especially of his linguistic behaviour, to determine which aspects of his unconscious mind can explain the symptoms considered to be abnormal. It is assumed that every aspect of behaviour is potentially significant (the notion of 'psychic determinism'—hence the everyday concept of 'Freudian slips'). The role of the unconscious is considered crucial, especially in providing us with motives for our behaviour. And the role of early childhood experience is held to be equally explanatory.

These aspects of psychiatry have often aroused controversy, because of the difficulty of proving to the sceptical observer that progress has been made, or that the progress, if made, has been due to the therapy.[14] It is difficult to see how one could formally evaluate the method, in any case, because of the difficulty of setting up controlled conditions for descriptive or experimental studies. It is its focus on the individual, and the personal rapport between patient and psychiatrist, which constitutes the method's strength and also its weakness. Indeed, the whole of psychiatry has come under attack in recent years, especially in the work of the British psychiatrist R. D. Laing, whose notions of 'anti-psychiatry' reject current conceptions of mental illness and treatment, on the grounds that they offer unnecessary restrictiveness and potential harm to the disturbed individuals, and recommend the search for alternative philosophies of investigation (such as the potential of self-directing treatment programmes).

This section has focused on *cognitive* and *abnormal psychology*, as these constitute two of the most relevant contributory areas to language pathology. A third important area, *developmental psychology*, was introduced in Chapter 2 (p. 51). Aspects of the study of the physiological basis of behaviour (*physiological psychology*) and of the neurological basis of behaviour (*neuropsychology*) will be discussed below (as part of Step 2 in the communication chain). Of the other main branches of psychology (see Fig. 10), a comment should also be made concerning *social psychology*, the study of man's social behaviour, or interaction with others. This is a topic of considerable potential relevance to our subject, e.g. in relation to the social evaluation of abnormal language states (see p. 36), and in analysing the attitudes and roles of clinician and patient, or of patients in group therapy sessions; but its clinical application to language work has to date been extremely limited and speculative, and consequently this field will be only briefly referred to elsewhere in this book (see p. 180). Nor will detailed reference be made to the various areas of *applied psychology*—the study of practical human problems using the theories and methods of general

---

[14] The same difficulty faces any method of clinical intervention, of course. Speech therapists, for example, have to be just as much concerned with the validation of their procedures.

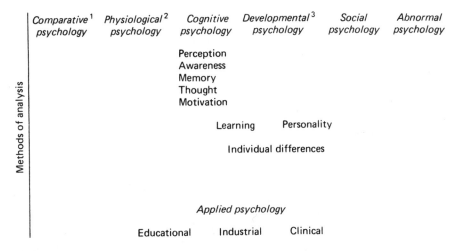

Fig. 10 The main branches of psychology
Notes: [1] see p. 63; [2] see p. 91; [3] see p. 51.

psychology. Particularly well-developed areas of application include *industrial psychology* (in relation to the health and efficiency of people at work), *educational psychology* (in relation to the health and efficiency of children in or preparing for school), and *clinical psychology* (in relation to mental health). Points of contact between the latter two applications and language pathology have already been referred to (p. 67); it should perhaps be noted in passing that there are points of contact with industrial psychology too, e.g. the effects of a noisy environment on hearing, or the provision of adequate facilities in the occupational rehabilitation of people with language problems. Finally, crosscutting all other classifications of psychological topics, is the area of *methodology*—the choice of methods of analysis for the investigation of any of the issues outlined in this section. The language pathologist needs to know about the different strengths and limitations of the many types of analytic method available to him: laboratory experimentation, field observation, surveys, tests, computer simulations, case histories (i.e. scientific biography of individuals being studied) and longitudinal studies (i.e. study of an individual through time)— the whole being underpinned by an awareness of (or, at least, an association with those who do have an awareness of) the complexities of experimental design and statistics. But these matters need proper introduction, as part of a psychologist's view of language pathology.[15]

[15] Further reading on psychology in general: E. R. Hilgard, R. C. Atkinson and R. L. Atkinson, *Introduction to psychology* (New York, Harcourt Brace Jovanovich, 5th edn, 1971), D. S. Wright, A. Taylor, D. R. Davies, W. Sluckin, S. G. M. Lee and J. T. Reason, *Introducing psychology: an experimental approach* (Harmondsworth, Penguin, 1970). On abnormal psychology etc., see: P. Hays (ed.), *New horizons in psychiatry* (Harmondsworth, Penguin, 2nd edn, 1971), I. G. Sarason, *Abnormal psychology: the problem of maladaptive behavior* (Englewood Cliffs, NJ, Prentice-Hall, 2nd edn, 1976), B. Maher, *Principles of psychopathology: an experimental approach* (New York, McGraw-Hill 1966).

Step 2　Neurological encoding

However the cognitive-linguistic basis of communication is organized by the brain, one thing is clear: ultimately, the information must be encoded into signals capable of being transmitted by the nervous system. It is a process which starts in the brain and then extends beyond it, as the signals are transmitted to their relevant destinations—the muscles and other variables which govern the production of our speech, writing or signing behaviour. It is therefore essential to know at least in outline what the body has available to enable this transmission of information to proceed, and to understand the main principles governing the process. The relevant disciplines are *neuroanatomy* and *neurophysiology*, from which the following perspective derives.[16]

The network of connections whereby signals (about the internal state of the body or its response to the environment) can be transmitted from one part of the body to another is known as the *nervous system*. It has been estimated that the system contains some 10 billion nerve cells. A nerve cell is known as a *neurone*, or *neuron* (both spellings are in current use), and its function is to conduct electrical impulses. The structure of the neurone is illustrated in Fig. 11. Each neurone has two main constituents: a cell body (sometimes called the soma, or cyton), which contains the nucleus of the cell; and one or more branching processes,[17] which conduct impulses to and from the cell body. These processes are what are generally referred to as *nerve fibres*; they vary in length from a few thousandths of a millimetre (or micron) to over a metre, the longest connecting the spinal cord to the extremities of the hands and feet. One process conducts impulses away from the cell body: this is known as the *axon*, which is readily identified by its relative lack of branches along most of its length. The other processes conduct impulses into the cell body: these are usually several in number, much shorter than the axon, and containing several branches; these processes are known as *dendrites*. The type of neurone illustrated in Fig. 11 is one which constitutes the majority in the nervous system (it is known as a 'multipolar' neurone); several other types of neurone exist, but the distinctions are not important for present purposes.

The direction in which impulses flow provides the basis for central binary classification of neurones into motor and sensory types. *Motor neurones* (or *motor nerves*) carry signals *away from* the cell body (i.e. they are 'efferent' nerves)[18] either to muscles which they cause to contract, or to glands which they cause to secrete. Muscles and glands are *effector organs*—they produce the effective end result of nerve impulses. *Sensory neurones* (or *sensory nerves*), by contrast, carry signals from 'receptor' nerve-endings in the skin

[16] Introductory accounts can be found in G. A. G. Mitchell, *The essentials of neuroanatomy* (Edinburgh and London, Churchill Livingstone 1973), E. R. Bickerstaff, *Neurology for nurses* (London, Hodder & Stoughton, 2nd edn, 1971), J. N. Walton, *Essentials of neurology* (London, Pitman, 4th edn, 1975). For a fuller account, see E. L. House and B. Pansky, *A functional approach to neuroanatomy* (New York, McGraw-Hill, 2nd edn, 1967).

[17] 'Process' is an anatomical term for any prominence or outgrowth from a central area.

[18] From the Latin, *e+fero*, 'to carry away from'; cf. below *ad+fero*, 'to carry towards'.

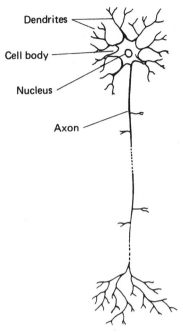

Fig. 11 Structure of the neurone

and other tissues, which respond to different stimuli (pain, touch, temperature etc.), *into* the cell body (i.e. they are 'afferent' nerves). One sequence of neurones transmits a signal from receptors to the brain; another sequence transmits signals in the reverse direction. The neurones connect at junctions known as *synapses* (sing. *synapse*/ˈsaɪnæps/): a neurone is said to synapse with another neurone, or with a receptor cell, or with an effector cell (such as a muscle fibre). According to the classical theory of neuronal transmission, the nerve impulse is conducted from neurone to neurone by chemical means—the impulse reaches the terminal branches of an axon and forces the release of chemical substances which provide a link between the axon and the dendrites or cell bodies of adjacent neurones. Many neurones in this way make synaptic contact with several thousand others.

The electrochemical impulses last for about a thousandth of a second. The speech at which they travel along the neurone is very variable—some impulses travel at less than a metre a second; others are much faster, reaching speeds of around 100 metres a second. The factors which govern the rate of impulse transmission are several—the type of fibre involved, its general environment, and above all the nature of its protective covering. Most fibres are covered in a white, fatty substance called *myelin*; the covering as a whole is referred to as a 'myelin sheath'. The sheath is about one millionth of a centimetre thick, and acts as an insulator for the fibre.

However, this surface covering is not total: every half millimetre or so the covering is broken, at points known as 'nodes of Ranvier' (after the French pathologist, Louis-Antoine Ranvier (1835–1922)), and there are also variations in the thickness of the sheath along different fibres. The significance of this is that the presence of myelin affects the rate at which impulses travel: the greater the distance between the nodes, the faster the rate of transmission; also, the thicker the fibres, the faster the rate of transmission. Moreover, nerves develop their myelin sheaths (or become 'myelinated') at different periods in human development. All fibres are 'unmyelinated' to begin with; the process of myelination continues until well after birth, and proves to be an important factor in the extent to which the nervous system is capable of transmitting efficiently several of the more complex voluntary movements. For example, it is possible that the relatively late appearance of certain types of sound in speech (e.g. with high acoustic frequency, such as [s]) may be due to the degree of myelination of the auditory nerve and the cortical areas to which it connects (see further below), this controlling the ability of the child to discriminate these sounds auditorily.[19] It should also be noted that there are a range of diseases which specifically affect myelin, the most well-known of these 'demyelinating diseases' being *disseminated (multiple) sclerosis*.

The 'nervous system', then, is the name given to the complex set of signal pathways through the body. Within this totality, a major division is made between the *central nervous system* (abbreviated to CNS) and the *peripheral nervous system*. In addition, a distinction is made between those aspects of the nervous system which are *somatic* (that is, concerned with the reception and transmission of stimuli to and from our sense organs) and those which are *autonomic* (that is, concerned with the involuntary, unconscious activities of the body, such as the regulation of blood pressure). However, it is the division between central and peripheral, and the further divisions which can be made within these headings, which provides the most relevant context for the classification of linguistic disability.

Central nervous system The CNS lies along the vertical axis of the body, and consists of the brain, the spinal cord, which connects to it, and their associated membranes, fluids and blood vessels. It is the complexity and potential of this system which needs to be appreciated. The average brain, weighing between 1300 grams (for females) and 1400 grams (for males), is only 2 per cent of body weight. But it contains some 5 million nerve cells per cubic centimetre—perhaps 2500 million cells in all. Moreover, we have already seen that synaptic interconnections may number several thousand, each in principle capable of transmitting a specific kind of information. The spinal cord is the elongated cylindrical part of the system which extends for some 45 cm into the vertebral column. The relationship of brain to spinal cord is illustrated in Figure 12.

---

[19] The point is argued in P. H. & M. W. Salus, 'Developmental neurophysiology and phonological acquisition order', *Language* **50** (1974), pp. 151–60.

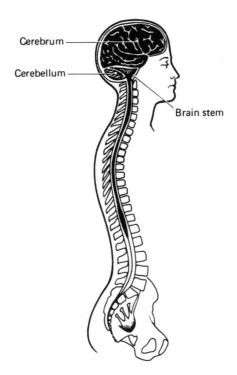

Fig. 12 The brain and spinal cord

Peripheral nervous system As its name suggests, this system of nerves links the CNS with the rest of the body, serving the parts in or near the body surface. Peripheral nerves which leave the spinal cord are known as *spinal nerves*. There are in fact 31 pairs of spinal nerves, each pair leaving the spinal cord at the level of each vertebra. In many respects more important for the study of communication is a second category of peripheral nerve: known as the *cranial nerves*, their role is to link the brain with the head and neck (the *cranium* is that part of the skull which encloses the brain). There are 12 cranial nerves, supplying the following areas:[20]

    I *Olfactory* nerve (sensory), from the nose
   II *Optic* nerve (sensory), from the eye
  III *Oculomotor* nerve (motor), supplying certain muscles of the eye
  IV *Trochlear* nerve (motor), supplying certain muscles of the eye
   V *Trigeminal* nerve (mixed, i.e. motor and sensory), motor to muscles of mastication and sensory to the face and tongue
  VI *Abducent* nerve (motor), supplying certain muscles of the eye
 VII *Facial* nerve (mixed), supplying all muscles of the face

[20] It is conventional to use roman numerals in listing the cranial nerves—referring to the VIth nerve, the XIIth nerve etc. The many kinds of interconnection between the cranial nerves are not given in the list.

VIII *Acoustic, auditory*, or *vestibulocochlear* nerve (sensory), from the ear
  IX *Glossopharyngeal* nerve (mixed), supplying the back of the tongue
      and the throat
   X *Vagus* nerve (mixed), motor to palate, pharynx and vocal cords;
      motor and sensory to organs of the chest and abdomen
  XI *Spinal* accessory nerve (motor), supplying certain shoulder muscles
 XII *Hypoglossal* nerve (motor), supplying the muscles of the tongue

It should thus be apparent that damage to the V, VII, VIII, IX, X, XI and XII nerves will have direct consequences on our language abilities, as will, less directly, damage to the set of nerves governing eye function.

We now need to proceed to a more detailed study of the brain, as in Chapter 4 we shall be referring to several categories of disability which are the result of damage to specific brain areas. But it will be useful, first, to introduce a terminological preliminary. In order to describe any area of human anatomy, it is necessary to use a terminology about which there is universal agreement, otherwise there would be ambiguity in knowing which specific part of the brain, for example, was being referred to. What would 'on the left side' mean, for instance? 'Left', from the point of view of the observer, or the person whose brain it is? To avoid such problems, it is conventional to see the human body as capable of being divided along various lines, or *planes*. Thus, we can imagine a line vertically dividing the front part of the body from the back part, as in Figure 13(a) below: this is known as the *coronal*, or *frontal* plane; and it divides the body into *anterior*, or *ventral* (i.e. front) and *posterior*, or *dorsal* (i.e. back) parts. Secondly, we can imagine the body being divided vertically into left and right sides, as in Figure 13(b): this is known as the *sagittal* plane; and if the division has been made exactly in the middle (in the *midline*, or *median*), it is referred to as the *medial sagittal* plane. *Lateral* refers to a plane further away from the midline; *medial* to a plane closer to the mid-line. The terms *left* and *right* are always used from the point of view of the body being described, and not as from the observer. Thirdly, we can imagine a line dividing the body horizontally, at right angles to its vertical axis, as in Figure 13(c): this is referred to as a *transverse*, or horizontal plane. Fourthly, relative position on the vertical axis is referred to using the terms *superior* (for higher up) and *inferior* (for lower down). Fifthly, a view of the body from underneath, looking upwards, is referred to as a *basal* view: see Fig. 13(d).

Using this terminology, we can now begin to identify those areas of the brain which are of particular importance for the study of linguistic disability. A general point to be made, first of all, is that the brain is not a single, undifferentiated structure, but contains several anatomically distinct regions. The largest part of the brain is known as the *cerebrum* (cf. Fig. 12). Its most noticeable feature is the way it is divided sagittally into two great lobes of similar size, the *cerebral hemispheres*. There is, accordingly, a *left hemisphere* and a *right hemisphere*, the differential function of which we shall

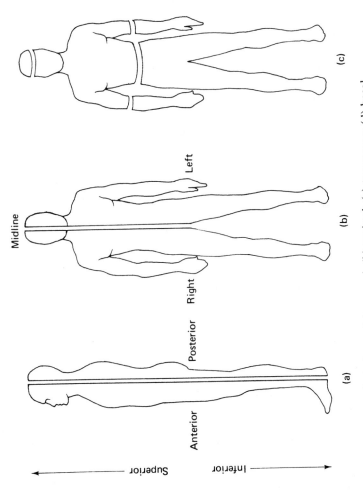

Fig. 13 Anatomical planes: (a) coronal; (b) sagittal; (c) transverse; (d) basal

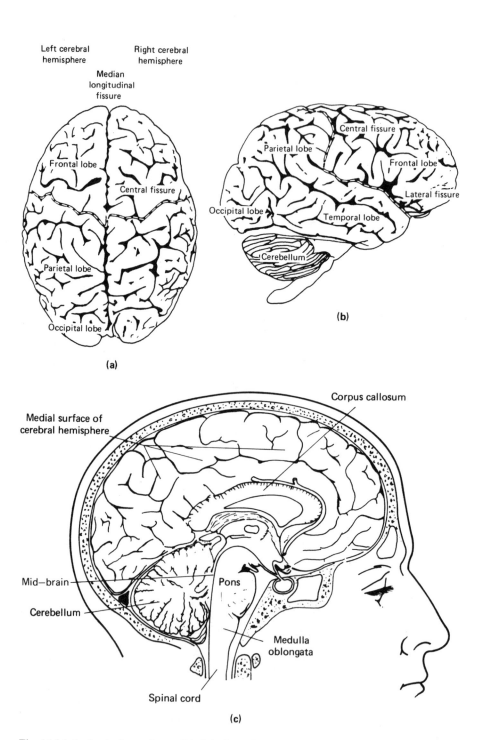

Fig. 14 (a) the brain from above; (b) right lateral view; (c) relationship between the main brain structures

discuss below. Each hemisphere has a rounded lateral surface, a flat medial surface where it lies against its fellow (see Fig. 14(c)), and an irregularly lobed inferior surface. Beneath the hemispheres is a thumb-sized midline structure, the *brain stem*, which connects the two hemispheres to the spinal cord. It is described as having three parts: the *midbrain* (from which the hemispheres spring), the *pons*, and the *medulla oblongata*, which continues below as the spinal cord. Arising dorsally from the pons is another major structure, the *cerebellum*, which is responsible for the maintenance of body posture and the smooth coordination of all movements, including walking and speaking. Buried deep within the hemispheres are further masses of nerve tissue, the *basal ganglia* (which help to control movement) and the *thalamus* (which relays and helps to analyse sensory information). The relationship between the hemispheres is shown from above in Fig. 14(a), laterally in Fig. 14(b), and that between the other structures is shown in medial sagittal section in Fig. 14(c).

The majority of research has been focused on the structure and function of the cerebrum, and in particular on its surface layer of grey matter (grey, because the cell bodies of the cerebral neurones are concentrated here) known as the cerebral *cortex*. The reason for this emphasis is that the cortex is the part of the brain which seems to be primarily involved in the decoding of information from the senses and in the control of voluntary movement and intellectual functions. It is also the area of the brain most amenable to direct observation and investigation. It contains about 14 billion cells and some 200 million fibre processes. Beneath the cortex is a body of white matter (white, because it is myelinated fibre), which transmits signals between cortex and brain stem, and from one area of the cortex to another. The most noticeable feature of the cortex is its lack of a smooth surface: what has happened is that, during its course of development (from between the third and fourth months of life in the womb) the surface of the brain has folded in upon itself along certain genetically predetermined lines. A large area of cortical tissue is thus packed into a relatively small anatomical space. The various folds that have been produced are known as *convolutions*, or *gyri* (singular: *gyrus*). The furrows on either side of the gyri are known as *sulci* (singular: *sulcus*). Each has a precise anatomical designation, but for present purposes we need concern ourselves only with the most dominant features, and those which are most relevant for language.

The brain is most commonly represented diagrammatically from above and laterally. The former view has been given in Figure 14(a); a lateral view (left lateral) is given in Figure 15. The dominant feature of the former view is the deep fissure, known as the *median longitudinal fissure*, which separates the hemispheres. It does not however extend the whole way down through the cerebrum; the two hemispheres are in fact joined deep within the cerebrum by a thick bundle of nerve fibres, known as the *corpus callosum*—see Figure 14(c)—the means whereby information from one hemisphere can be transmitted to the other. The dominant features of the

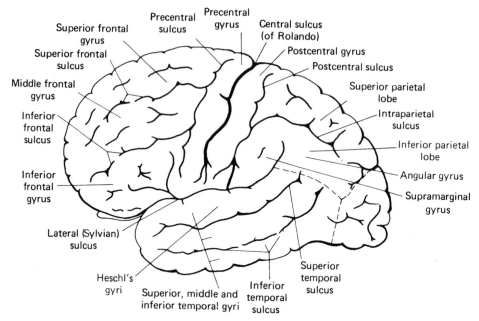

Fig. 15 Superolateral surface of cerebral hemisphere

lateral view are also fissures, or sulci:[21] the *central sulcus*, or *fissure of Rolando* (named after the Italian anatomist, Luigi Rolando (1773–1831), and the *lateral sulcus*, or *Sylvian fissure* (after the Flemish anatomist, François de la Boë Sylvius (1614–72)). These fissures are of particular importance, because they are used as the primary anatomical basis for dividing the brain up into different major areas, or *lobes*. Four such lobes are universally recognized, within each hemisphere, based on the topographical relation of these areas to the skull (the temporal lobe corresponds to the temporal bone, etc.):

(a) the *frontal* lobe—from the front of the brain above the Sylvian fissure and extending as far back as the fissure of Rolando. The frontal lobe is crossed by three main sulci (superior, inferior and precentral), and four main gyri (superior, middle, inferior and precentral).

(b) the *temporal* lobe—the area beneath the Sylvian fissure, extending posteriorly until the junction with the occipital lobe. It is crossed by two main sulci (superior and inferior) and three main gyri (superior, middle and inferior).

(c) the *parietal* lobe (pronounced /pə'raɪətəl/)—extending from behind the fissure of Rolando to the occipital lobe. It is crossed by two main sulci (postcentral and intraparietal) and three main gyri (superior, inferior and postcentral).

[21] 'Sulcus' is the more general term. Originally, the difference was that a sulcus was a relatively shallow furrow in the surface of the hemisphere, whereas a fissure was much deeper.

(d) the *occipital* lobe (pronounced /ɒk'sɪpɪtəl/)—a relatively small lobe in the most posterior part of the cerebrum. Its anterior boundary, seen on the medial surface, is the parieto-occipital sulcus, and the main sulci are the calcarine and post-calcarine sulci, also on the flat medial surface. On the lateral surface, this lobe merges with the parietal lobe.
These are all indicated in Fig. 15.

The significance of these identifications resides in the possibility that different functions can be associated with the different lobes. For example, the anterior part of the frontal lobes has been traditionally associated with the development of personality type and abstract thought. The occipital lobe is associated with visual processing. Probably the most important functional distinctions, from the viewpoint of this book, are those which have been drawn in relation to the parts of the cortex on either side of the fissure of Rolando, as this is where the fundamental medical and behavioural division into motor and sensory modes of operation seems primarily to reside. This operational distinction has already been drawn in our earlier discussion of types of neurone, but we now need to extend it to the study of the general properties of the nervous system. Indeed, the motor/sensory distinction was one of the earliest findings of neurological studies of the brain. It was shown that there was a stateable relationship between voluntary body movements (summarized under the heading of *motor* activities) and the part of the cortex immediately anterior to the Rolandic fissure. Electrical stimulation of a specific part of this region would produce a regular movement in a specific part of the body. It emerged that the body's motor activities were represented in this part of the brain in an 'upside-down' order: the uppermost part of the region seemed to control the legs, and the lowest part the face. The region as a whole was accordingly referred to as the *motor cortex*. A common way of representing the relationship is to draw the 'motor homunculus'—an invention of the American neurologist, Wilder Graves Penfield.[22] This is a figure of a human form in which the size of the parts of the body is made proportional to the extent of the brain area which is involved with them: see Fig. 16(a). Notice the large area serving the muscles of the hand (especially the thumb), the face, the tongue and the eye muscles. What is also important to note, in passing, is that the motor cortex in each hemisphere controls the movements on the *opposite* side of the body. This is because the bundles (or 'tracts') of nerve fibres from the motor cortex, known as the *pyramidal tracts*, cross over each other on their way down through the brain stem, when they reach the medulla oblongata. The phenomenon is referred to as the 'crossing' or 'decussation' of the pyramids. It is this which accounts for the fact that brain damage to one hemisphere is correlated with bodily effects, such as paralysis, on the opposite (or *contralateral*) side.

The correlative area of the brain, lying immediately posterior to the

[22] See, for example, W. G. Penfield and L. Roberts, *Speech and brain mechanisms* (Princeton, NJ, Princeton University Press 1959).

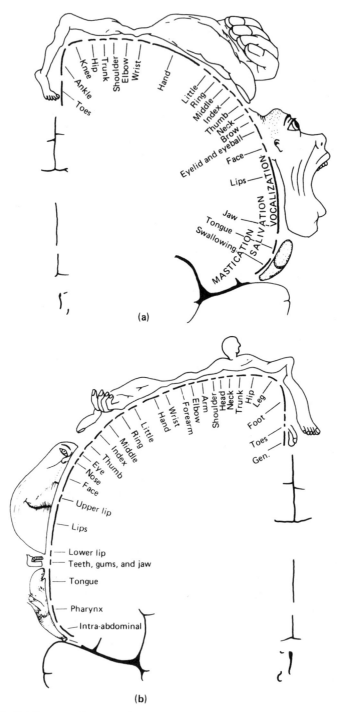

Fig. 16 (a) Penfield's motor homunculus; (b) Penfield's sensory homunculus

Rolandic fissure, is the part which deals with the reception and interpretation of incoming stimuli. The general term here is *sensory*: one refers to the *sensory cortex*, for which a 'sensory homunculus' has likewise been drawn: see Fig. 16(b). Notice here the large area devoted to the skin of the fingertips, the mouth area and tongue, and the tiny area given to the skin of the trunk.

Similar *localizations* of function have been proposed for other lobes and parts of the brain. From the linguistic point of view, it is important to note the areas which have been proposed for the processing of speech, listening, reading and writing. These are mainly located at or around the junction between the frontal, parietal and temporal lobes, as can be seen from Figure 17. The numbers in this figure derive from the work of the German neurologist Karl Brodmann (1868–1918) who in 1909 made a detailed classification of the areas of the cortex, based upon the cellular differences observed (a 'cyto-architectonic' classification). The relevant 'Brodmann areas' for language are, accordingly:

1–3, in the anterior part of the parietal lobe; these are the primary areas involved with the processing of sensation, and may be connected with the speech and auditory areas (see below) at a deeper cortical level, as they will provide feedback concerning the parts of the vocal apparatus involved;

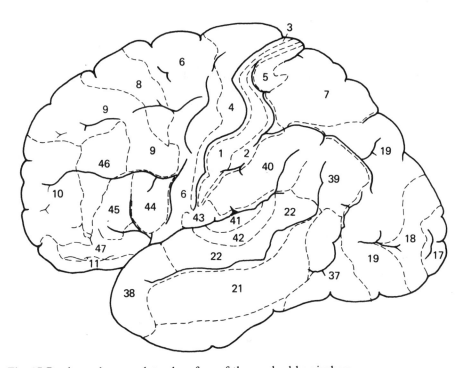

Fig. 17 Brodmann's superolateral surface of the cerebral hemisphere

similarly, area 4, in front of the Rolandic fissure, will contain information about the motor functioning of the speech/writing apparatus.

17, in the occipital lobe, is the primary area concerned with visual reception and processing, and is thus of importance for reading and writing.

39, 40 and much of 22, in the superior temporal gyrus, extending into the angular and supramarginal gyri; this is generally known as 'Wernicke's area', after the German neurologist Karl Wernicke (1848–1905), though its precise extent is disputed; its main function seems to be the comprehension of speech, but other functions have been noted; area 39, the angular gyrus, forming the posterior part of the inferior parietal lobe, lies between the auditory and visual association areas, and seems critical for the processing of written symbols.

9, in the posterior part of the middle frontal gyrus; this area is known as 'Exner's centre' (after the German neurologist, S. Exner, who postulated this area for the motor control of writing, in 1881).

41, 42 transverse convolutions in the superior temporal gyrus; the main areas for auditory reception; also known as 'Heschl's gyri', after the Austrian pathologist R. L. Heschl (1824–81).

44, and part of 45, at the anterior end of the left inferior frontal gyrus; this area was first defined by the French neurologist Paul Pierre Broca (1824–80), and thereafter often referred to as 'Broca's area'; its main function seems to be the encoding of speech, and it is accordingly sometimes referred to as the 'motor speech area'.

As a consequence of this approach, each lobe can be associated with a set of 'typical' disorders, and this provides an important context for the study of linguistic disability. Patients with frontal lobe disorders, for example, display a range of personality and intellectual difficulties: aggression, antisocial behaviour and apathy, under the former heading; poor memory, learning and thinking, under the latter. There may be lack of emotional control or sense of appropriateness. If there are lesions[23] of the motor cortex, there will be a loss of voluntary movement (but not autonomic or reflex movements) in the area involved on the contralateral side. The most important concepts to know here are those involved in the classification of paralysis (though it should be noted that the distinction between *-paresis* and *-plegia* is not universally used):

hemiparesis a weakening of one body side (a 'paresis' is an incomplete loss of muscular power)
hemiplegia a paralysis of one body side
monoplegia a paralysis of one limb
quadriplegia a paralysis of all four limbs
paraplegia a paralysis of both legs

Damage to the sensory cortex in the parietal lobe will cause loss of

---

[23] A *lesion* is an area of tissue whose structure or function has been altered or destroyed due to injury or disease.

discrimination: the subject will be aware of a sensation, such as a touch, but will be unable to locate it on his body. He can still feel pain, which is appreciated at thalamic level, but will be unable to define its site. *Hemianaesthesia*—loss of sensation in one side of the body—only occurs along with damage at a lower level (e.g. in the brain stem). Lesions further back in the parietal lobe cause inability to orientate spatially, or to recognize objects by touch (*astereognosis*). In some cases, the patient may no longer recognize the limb involved as belonging to him, and disregard it—for instance, while dressing.

Lesions in the temporal lobe will, as we have seen, be likely to affect speech, and memory; smell and taste are also often affected. Occipital lesions will primarily affect vision, producing a range of problems which the language pathologist must be aware of, if he wishes to understand the patient's difficulties with reading and writing—and also with speech comprehension.[24] The main categories we need to be aware of are:

hemianopia—loss of vision in one half of the visual field; subdivided into *right hemianopia* (the right-hand side of the visual field is affected) and *left hemianopia* (the left-hand side of the visual field is affected)
homonymous—the corresponding parts of the two eyes
scotoma (plural *scotomata*)—loss of vision in the centre of the visual field
quadrantic—a quarter segment of the visual field

Thus, for example, a patient with a 'right homonymous hemianopia' (one of the commonest patterns encountered in language pathology, because of its association with left hemisphere damage to speech) would have a visual field which could be drawn thus:

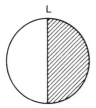 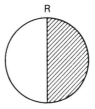

The patient is unable to see anything which falls within the scope of his visual field on the right-hand side, in either eye. Lastly, a frequent feature of cortical damage is a tendency for the patient to accept blandly, disregard or even deny his disability.

There is, then, a range of disorders that can be associated, fairly directly, with damage to specific areas of the brain. But how is this damage caused?

---

[24] Vision is an important factor in establishing comprehension of speech. To ask someone to name what is in a picture makes sense only if the person can see the part of the picture you are referring to. In cases where the patient may not reply to your question, this could be due either to his inability to understand what you are saying, or to his inability to see what you are referring to, or of course a mixture of both problems.

The whole range of diseases classified in Chapter 2 (pp. 21–2) is relevant, but I will refer here only to the categories which turn up most frequently in discussing the etiology of linguistic pathology. Perhaps the most important point to bear in mind is the total dependence of the brain on its blood supply, and the oxygen this conveys. While the brain may constitute only 2 per cent of a person's body weight, it consumes 25 per cent of the body's oxygen intake when at rest. If deprived of oxygen for more than three minutes at normal temperatures, the brain cells die. Consequently, any diminution in the blood supply (or *ischemia*) to an area of the brain will lead to the pathological death of cells (or *necrosis*). Medical textbooks will refer to *ischemic necrosis* (or *infarction*) of the brain area supplied by the occluded (i.e. blocked) vessel. It is important to stress that there is no recovery possible in the affected (or 'infarcted') area.

The blood supply to the brain is illustrated in Fig. 18. It is carried by two pairs of arteries:

1 the internal *carotid* arteries, which pass through the petrous bone in the base of the skull and divide into the *anterior cerebral arteries*, which supply much of the medial surface of the hemispheres, and the large *medial cerebral arteries*, which supply much of the lateral surface of the hemispheres;

2 the *vertebral* arteries, which pass along bony channels in the cervical vertebrae, join to form a single *basilar* artery which lies on and supplies the brain stem and cerebellum, and then redivide to form the *posterior cerebral arteries*, supplying the occipital lobes and parts of adjoining areas. The two systems are not isolated, however: the carotid and vertebral systems are joined by *communicating arteries*, to produce a complete circle of blood vessels on the inferior surface of the hemispheres. This is known as the *circle of Willis* (after the British physician Thomas Willis (1621–75), whose major work on the anatomy of the brain, *Cerebri anatome*, was published in 1664). The significance of this is that the pressure of the blood in all four arterial systems is kept equal at all times, and that any area of the brain can obtain a supply from different sources, if one artery becomes damaged.

The most common types of linguistic pathology result from *cerebro-vascular accidents* (CVAs), generally known as *strokes*. The 'accident' refers to the cell damage which takes place as a result of reduced oxygen supply. There may be several reasons for this. The commonest is that due to *atherosclerosis*. In adult Western man, all large arteries tend to become 'furred up' with fatty cholesterol deposits called *atheroma* (from the Greek word for 'porridge'), particularly in the carotid arteries, the coronary arteries of the heart muscle, and the leg arteries. This is associated principally with smoking, high blood pressure, diet and lack of exercise. The deposits cause narrowing (*stenosis*) within the arteries, and a clot of blood (*thrombus*) may form on the patches, or plaques, of atheroma (*thrombosis*), causing sudden complete obstruction. If for any reason the blood pressure should fall (as in a mild heart attack), then the previously poor flow through a narrowed artery may become completely inadequate. Foreign matter may enter the blood stream at some point (e.g. a blood clot, piece of tissue, piece of bullet) and travel along it until it reaches the cerebral arteries, where it may lodge; the piece of foreign matter is known as an *embolus*, and the resulting situation is an *embolism*. An artery may rupture (*haemorrhage*) in

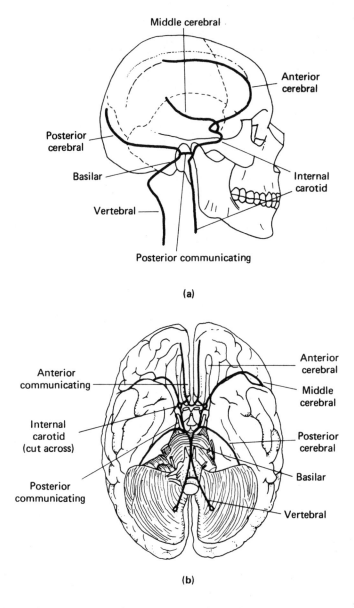

Fig. 18 (a) lateral view of the arteries supplying the brain; (b) basal view of the arteries supplying the brain

various ways. If for example there is a defect in the arterial wall, the artery will swell with blood at that point, to produce an *aneurysm*, which may subsequently haemorrhage (usually, as a sub-arachnoid haemorrhage). Some unfortunate people are born with small weak areas in their cerebral arteries, often near the circle of Willis, and develop 'berry aneurysms' in early adult life. The result of all these conditions is a CVA, usually referred to as a 'left CVA' or a 'right CVA', depending on the hemisphere affected, and generally associated with a contralateral paralysis.

But CVAs are not the only factors which cause brain damage. Genetic diseases can affect the brain: an example is the interference with the neural development of the nervous system which produces spina bifida. Then there are the many kinds of abnormal cell growth in the brain, resulting in intracranial tumours. Several types of infectious disease affect the brain, such as meningitis (the inflammation of the membraneous covering of the brain and spinal cord) or poliomyelitis (the inflammation of the grey matter of the spinal cord). And there is the important category of traumatic damage. Birth injury, for example, can cause direct brain trauma by bruising and bleeding within the soft infant skull, or by reduced oxygen supply during a prolonged delivery, producing cerebral palsy. There are also the injuries due to headwounds, as in war-time, car accidents, falls, and so on. A very wide range of factors is involved in the investigation of brain damage. What is unclear, in our present state of knowledge, is whether there is any predictable relationship between brain damage due to one or other of these factors and the linguistic behaviour manifested by the patient. The location and severity of the damage will obviously be controlling factors, but it is difficult to be precise because so often it is unclear how much of the brain has been affected. New techniques of brain scanning (such as the technique developed in the 1970s by the firm of EMI, and known as computerized axial tomography, or CAT scanning) have helped enormously in this respect, but there is still a great gap between the gross behavioural observations which can be made related to brain-scan data, and the fine behavioural observations used in linguistic investigations, with which brain-scan data cannot yet usefully be correlated.

Lastly, in relation to neurological encoding and transmission, due attention should be paid to the way the motor/sensory distinction is maintained throughout the body. In particular, from the viewpoint of speech and writing disorders, the further classification of disorders affecting the motor systems of nerves needs to be mentioned. It will be recalled that the pyramidal tracts convey impulses from the motor cortex (and from certain other parts of the brain) into the brain stem and spinal cord. The neurones involved in this 'first stage of the journey' are collectively referred to as the *upper motor neurones*. Where they end, new neurones begin, which take the impulses to other parts of the body, via the peripheral nerve system. These neurones are collectively labelled *lower motor neurones*. They are affected in fact not only by the impulses from the pyramidal fibres, but also by other parts of the nervous system. At the end of the lower motor neurones are the effector organs—the points of neuromuscular junction where nerve impulses are turned into physiological movement (the specific study of neurophysiology). The importance of these distinctions is that they are used as the basis for a classification of disease which has major implications for speech and writing.

Disease may affect motor neurones selectively. *Motor neurone disease*, a rare degenerative disease which is slowly progressive and ultimately fatal, can attack the upper or the lower motor neurones. For example, upper motor neurone (UMN) disease affects the brain stem in bulbar palsy, and in pseudo-bulbar palsy,[25] producing weakness, wasting and twitching of the muscles of the face, palate and tongue (with consequent problems of swallowing and speaking). A similar muscular deterioration may be seen in lower motor neurone (LMN) disease, with muscles displaying decreased tone,[26] and decreased or absent reflexes. Poliomyelitis, a viral disease, attacks lower motor neurones alone in the brain stem and spinal cord, causing paralysis and wasting of muscles. The peripheral nerves may be damaged (for instance, cut or crushed in accidents) or be involved by tumours (as when there is paralysis of the nerves to the vocal cords in lung cancer). They may be involved in wasting diseases (polyneuritis) or damaged by viruses, as in the facial weaknesses of Bell's palsy. Finally, at the points of neuromuscular junction, disease may affect the ability of the muscle to respond to nerve impulses. For example, there may be a rapid loss of power in muscle contraction, as is characteristic of myasthenia gravis: the muscular fatigue produces increasing faintness and slurring of speech, amongst other things.

These are some of the main medical points which a language pathologist needs to be aware of in order to appreciate the condition of the patient he is studying. The above perspective, it should also be emphasized, is in its barest outline, and should be supplemented directly with specialized reading on the main issues.[27] There are also two points of a general nature to be made, concerning the whole process of reasoning involved in this part of the book: one concerns the notion of localization, the other the notion of laterality.

[25] The 'bulb' is the old name for the medulla oblongata. In bulbar palsy, there is disease at some point along the cranial nerve pathways whose motor nuclei are in the medulla, thus producing a weakness and deterioration in the muscles supplied by those nerves. 'Pseudo-bulbar palsy' is so-called because the clinical signs resemble those of bulbar palsy, though in fact their origin is different, stemming from above the medulla (as is better reflected in the alternative name for this disorder, 'supra-bulbar' palsy). The term palsy is used in place of the more general term 'paralysis', when one is talking about a specific type of paralysis in the context of a specific disorder.

[26] 'Muscle tone' refers to the normal state of tension of a muscle. Poor (or 'flaccid') muscle tone in LMN disease contrasts with the increased muscle tone of UMN disease, the latter accounting for the muscular spasms characteristic of certain kinds of spasticity.

[27] For example, M. L. E. Espir and F. C. Rose, *The basic neurology of speech* (Oxford, Blackwell, 2nd edn, 1976), and I. T. Draper, *Lecture notes on neurology* (Oxford, Blackwell, 4th edn, 1974), both of which provide an account of neuropathology. A standard text is W. B. Matthews and H. Miller, *Diseases of the nervous system* (Oxford, Blackwell, 2nd edn, 1975).

Localization

The idea that a single area of the brain can be related to a single bodily activity, or function, such as memory, vision, emotion, speech, or, more specifically, tongue, finger or leg control, is known as 'localization theory' (or the theory of cerebral localization). The claims of this theory have been controversial for over a century. In its extreme form, the theory states that there is a strict one-to-one relationship between the anatomical areas of the brain and bodily function. In this form, it derives from the views of Broca, first formulated in 1861 with reference to speech, and later extended to cover other functions. From the earliest years, however, counter-evidence to this strict form of the hypothesis was forthcoming (prominent opponents included the British neurologists Hughlings Jackson and Henry Head). With an apparently undamaged Broca's area, for example, a patient would still manifest disordered speech; and conversely, damage to Broca's area would not inevitably, and to the same degree, cause speech problems. As Jackson put it: 'to locate the damage which destroys speech, and to locate speech, are two different things.' It was evident that conclusions could not be drawn based solely on observation of the cortex: concentrating on the surface area of the brain ignored the possibility that at a deeper, 'subcortical' level, associations might be available between one area and another, and perhaps between the hemispheres (via the corpus callosum) which would continue to facilitate the activity being monitored. In fact, brain research continues to demonstrate the importance of these subcortical areas within the cerebrum, and also of those parts of the brain other than the cerebrum, in explaining the basis of behaviour. For instance, speech production is these days discussed not only with reference to Broca's area, but also with reference to several other parts of the cortex, and to such 'deeper' parts of the brain as the thalamus. But this is not to move to a theory of opposite extremes—that there is no localization at all, and that every main region of the brain is *equally* able to cope with a particular function, or that the whole of the brain is always involved in all activities (a theory of 'equipotentiality'). Rather, it is to argue for a midway position between the two extremes: it is allowed that certain areas of the brain are primarily involved in a particular function, but this must be seen in the context of the brain as a whole; that is, in certain circumstances other areas of the brain may become involved in that function, or even take over that function altogether. It is this possibility, indeed, that provides hope for those who work remedially with brain-damaged patients.

On this view, then, we are able to continue talking about the particular significance of an area such as Broca's for speech, but we must not conclude from this that the only function of this area is for speech, nor, conversely, that speech could not be mediated by other areas. A fuller account of this issue, within the field of neuropsychology, would provide many details of the kinds of interrelationships involved. But research in this area is inevitably a slow, intricate and often inconclusive process. The main problems are how to obtain information about the internal structure of the brain, and having obtained it, how to interpret it. There are three main techniques used in obtaining this information, and all present major methodological problems to the researcher. Firstly, we may simply monitor brain activity using *electroencephalography* (EEG), recording fluctuations in the brain's electrical potentials, temperature, or biochemistry while the brain is at rest and in response to different stimuli. The various traces obtained however produce an enormous amount of data, and present major problems of computational analysis. Secondly, we may excite an area of cortex exposed during surgery under local anaesthesia, in the conscious patient, and ask the patient what he feels (e.g. 'I can feel something touching my thumb') or observe his behaviour. This is not painful (the brain itself is insensitive!), and is a classical technique of brain study, being used in the establishment of the motor-sensory sites referred to above. But it is a technique which can be used only in a very limited way, for obvious reasons. Thirdly, we can examine the effect that brain lesions have on behaviour—correlating the person's performance with the location and severity of the lesion (Broca's original technique, supported by post-mortem analysis). The problems here relate to the difficulty in precisely estimating the area of brain damage (cf. above), and hitherto on the limited information available about the patient's behaviour 'before and after' the brain damage. As a consequence of the problems associated with each of these techniques, the relevant branches of contemporary psychology (neuropsychology, or physiological psychology) are inevitably more concerned with methodological issues than with providing alternative accounts of the brain as a whole. And in its experimental bias, it contrasts markedly with the investigative techniques of linguistics.[28]

Laterality
Caution also needs to be advocated in relation to the second main issue in the study of brain function—the question of hemispheric function. The most notable feature of the cerebrum, referred to above, is the way in which it is split into two main hemispheres, of roughly equal size and proportions (there are certain asymmetries between the hemispheres, but these need not concern us here). The question originally arose as to whether one hemisphere was more important than the other for the performance of body functions. It should be noted that this was a different issue from the question of localization discussed above: we are not here concerned about *where* in the hemisphere a function lies, but rather with whether a function is *only* to be found in one hemisphere. The earliest answer was that the dominant hemisphere was the left, in most people, and a correlation was asserted

[28] These issues are fully discussed in G. B. Milner, *Physiological psychology* (New York, Holt, Rinehart & Winston 1970) Ch. 1. For an introduction to neuropsychology, see A. R. Luria, *The working brain: an introduction to neuropsychology* (Harmondsworth, Penguin 1973), K. Walsh, *Neuropsychology* (London, Churchill Livingstone 1978).

between this and the fact that most people were also right-handed.[29] It was assumed that the left hemisphere was dominant in right-handed persons. In the minority of cases of left-handedness, accordingly, it was assumed that the opposite correlation applied—that these people would have a right hemispheric dominance for all body functions.

There have been several changes in these views over the years. No longer is it felt that a single hemisphere is *the* dominant one, for all functions. Rather, *each* hemisphere is seen as being dominant for certain functions and non-dominant for others. One hemisphere is said to be more dominant than the other for a particular function when it is more important than the other for the performance of that function. On this basis, we can accept the view, propounded by Broca and others, that the left hemisphere is dominant for speech (in right-handed people). Lesions of Broca's area in the left hemisphere do generally interfere with speech; whereas lesions in the corresponding area (the 'homologous' area) in the right hemisphere do not affect speech. Likewise, it can be shown that lesions of the left hemisphere produce disorders of reading and writing, loss of verbal memory, defects in right/left orientation, oversimplification and lack of detail in drawing, inability to perform certain kinds of purposeful movements, and so on. Similarly, lesions of the right hemisphere produce disorders of spatial orientation, recognition of faces and objects, certain emotional responses, grossly distorted drawing, and several other problems. Certain abilities seem to be represented in both hemispheres (e.g. musical abilities), but apart from these, it is possible to talk of the hemispheres being 'specialized' for the various functions listed. There are many areas of body function, however, where the question of dominance cannot be answered, in the present state of knowledge. Even in relation to language, there are uncertainties—for example, whether the whole of the non-segmental effects of language (cf. p. 41) are processed by the left hemisphere, or whether the right is also in some way involved.

As with localization theory above, a major problem is obtaining the information. The study of the effects of naturally-occurring lesions (as in strokes) has been the main source of information. Another results from the surgical removal of the cortical areas of a diseased hemisphere ('hemispherectomy'), or from temporarily anaesthetizing one hemisphere (for instance, by injecting sodium-amytal into the carotid artery); another results from the study of severely epileptic patients whose condition can be much improved by having their left hemisphere surgically separated from the right ('commisurotomy')—the so-called 'split-brain' studies.[30] A further source of information is the study of the varying brain waves in response to different stimuli, using the electroencephalograph. Other information comes from the study of medically normal persons, attempting to show from

[29] How dominance is established in the individual is unclear—whether it is a genetic or learned development (or some combination). The first signs of lateral preference in children may emerge as early as 9 months, but a definite pattern is unlikely until the third year.

[30] These are well reviewed in D. B. Fry, *Homo loquens* (Cambridge, CUP 1977), Ch. 9, and S. J. Dimond, *The double brain* (London, Churchill Livingstone 1972).

their varying reaction times to auditory, visual and tactile stimuli, presented first to one side of the body and then the other, whether one hemisphere is more effective in processing the stimuli. In a 'dichotic listening task', for instance, an auditory stimulus is played into one ear, and the time it takes for the person to respond to this stimulus is measured: we would expect language stimuli to be more rapidly processed by the left ear than by the right (in right-handed people), and this is generally what happens.

But the methodological and theoretical problems of doing research in this area are very great. It is always difficult drawing conclusions about a pathological population from a normal one, as we do not know whether other parts of the brain than those being medically investigated have also been affected and are thus producing abnormal responses. It is unclear how far it is possible to generalize about the performance of a single hemisphere following a hemispherectomy, for instance. And in the reaction-time experiments, it is difficult to keep the stimuli accurately graded, to control for variations in the subject's response, and to explain the variations in reaction-time which emerge. For instance, if a language signal is presented to the right ear, is the delay in reaction-time due to the time it takes for the signal to cross over to the left side, where it will be processed, or might not other factors have intervened, such as a change in the subject's attention?

One further finding needs to be referred to here, namely that the correlation between language dominance and handedness is not as symmetrical as was once thought. As we have seen, the left hemisphere is dominant in the vast majority (98 per cent) of right-handed people; but it also seems to be dominant in a significant proportion of left-handed people also (about 60 per cent). Aphasia (see p. 140) hardly ever occurs in right-handed people who have suffered right-hemisphere lesions; but left-handed people can become aphasic with lesions in either hemisphere, and a permanent effect is much more likely, also, if the lesion is on the left side. But here too a great deal of work remains to be done for the full complexity of this relationship to become clear. The notion of handedness is itself a complex one, despite the apparent simplicity of the distinction between left and right: whether we are left- or right-handed may depend on several factors (such as the level of complexity of the task being performed), and 'mixed' dominance is fairly common (e.g. we might be right-handed, but left-footed, or left-eyed). In investigating linguistic disability, therefore, deductions based on handedness have to be viewed with caution.[31]

Step 3 Anatomical-physiological encoding

It makes sense to take these two aspects of communication together, in continuing our detailed discussion of the communication chain. The physiology of speech is most clearly described at the same time as the

[31] These issues are reviewed in S. J. Dimond and J. G. Beaumont, *Hemisphere function in the human brain* (London, Elek 1974), esp. Chs. 2, 4, 5.

anatomy of the relevant speech organs. I shall in this section concentrate on speech, as it is here that the majority of the classificatory distinctions made in Chapter 4 take their rise. The best place to start is with a view of the vocal apparatus, or *vocal organs*, as a whole—that is, with those parts of the body that are involved in the production of speech. This is given in Fig. 19.

Perhaps the most notable feature of this diagram is the amount of the body which has to be included. People sometimes think of the vocal organs as being solely a matter of mouth and throat, but far more is plainly involved. The vocal organs include the *lungs*, *windpipe* (or *trachea*), the *larynx* (which contains the *vocal cords*), the *throat* (or *pharynx*), the *mouth* and the *nose*. The system of cavities above the larynx is known as the *vocal tract*, the shape of which can be altered to produce the various sounds of speech.

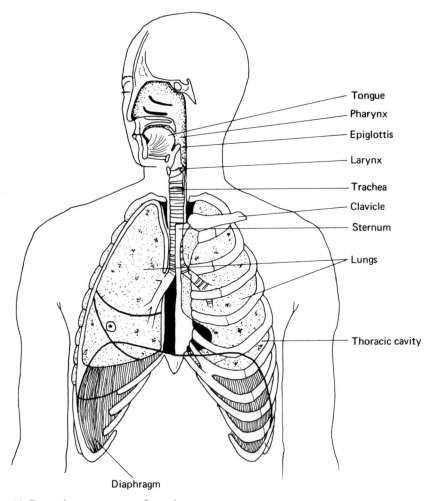

Fig. 19 General arrangement of vocal organs

But before any sound can be produced at all, there must be a source of energy. For speech, the energy takes the form of an air-stream which has been set in motion by the lungs. The air involved in the production of the majority of speech sounds is lung air (or *pulmonic* air) flowing outwards from the lungs (the direction is *egressive*). Occasionally in speech other air-stream mechanisms are used. For example, in making a *tut-tut* noise with our tongue, the sound produced is made without the help of lung air—as can be demonstrated by the fact that we can continue to breath in and out while making the noise. The source of energy in this case is within the mouth itself, arising from a sharp movement using the back of the tongue against the roof of the mouth (a *velaric* air-stream mechanism). It is also possible—though not very normal—to speak while the air-stream is flowing inwards towards the lungs (the direction is *ingressive*), as for example when we speak while out of breath. But for most practical purposes, in English, we can discuss speech production in terms of the use of pulmonic egressive air.

Speech is, then, 'superimposed' on the normal pattern of exhalation and inhalation—the *respiratory cycle*. But while speaking, this cycle changes from a pattern of equal duration for the two halves of this cycle to one where there is a rapid inhalation and a very slow exhalation. We normally breathe in about 20 times a minute, while at rest; but while speaking, our inhalations may reduce to less than 10 a minute. The respiratory cycle takes place through the action of the ribs and lungs, which constitute part of the *thoracic cavity*. When the volume of this cavity is increased, pressure within it drops, and air is sucked in from mouth and nose. Conversely, when the volume of this cavity is decreased, pressure is raised, and air is forced outwards. The changes in volume required are primarily the result of the movements of the ribs and sternum (or breastbone) and of the contraction of the *diaphragma* muscle (or *diaphragm*), which separates the lungs from the lower (abdominal) cavities. Several neck and shoulder muscles are also involved in helping to raise the thoracic cage; several muscles of the abdomen are also involved in the corresponding lowering process.

The air-stream from the lungs is normally inaudible. It is made audible when it is interfered with on its outward journey, the molecules of air being made to vibrate rapidly. The first place where this interference takes place is in the larynx, using the vocal cords (see Figure 20). The larynx, or 'voice box', is a casing of muscle and cartilage, about 8 cm by 5 cm, which at the front is most noticeable in the protruberance in the neck known as the *thyroid cartilage* (or 'Adam's apple'). Its functions are both biological and linguistic. Under the former heading, the larynx acts as a valve to shut off the lungs, e.g. to aid in the process of exertion, or to prevent foreign matter entering the trachea. Under the latter heading, the larynx is involved in the production of several types of sound effect, depending on the mode of action of the vocal cords.

The larynx consists basically of nine cartilages. Figure 20 shows the three most noticeable cartilages: the *thyroid*, the *cricoid* and, at the top, the pear-

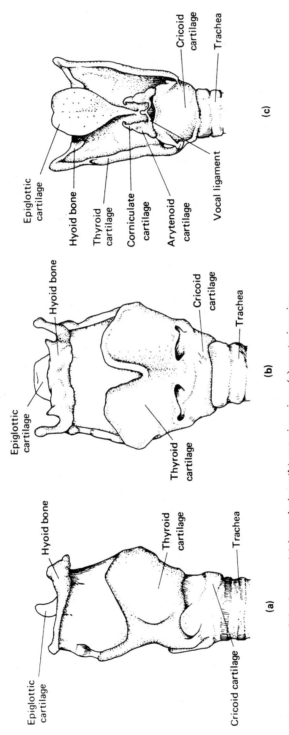

Fig. 20 Structure of the larynx: (a) lateral view; (b) anterior view; (c) posterior view

shaped *epiglottis* (which helps to cover the trachea while swallowing). The remaining six consist of three pairs of cartilages, visible in Figure 21: the *arytenoid*, the *corniculate* and the *cuneiform* cartilages. The cartilages are connected to each other by joints, around which they move in response to the pressures from the various muscles and ligaments to which they are attached. A very wide range of movements is possible, and this permits a correspondingly wide range of sound effects. Situated above the larynx is the *hyoid* bone, which acts as a base for the tongue, and which is also connected to the larynx by various muscles.

The vocal cords (sometimes called vocal 'folds' or 'bands') are two pearly white muscular folds running posteriorly from a single point at the anterior end of the thyroid cartilage to the anterior processes of the two arytenoid cartilages (see Figure 21). Their inner edge is about 23 mm in men, and about 18 mm in women. The space between them is known as the *glottis*. It is about 12 mm wide at its widest point when fully open. The extent of the glottal opening, and also the degree and kind of tension affecting the vocal cords, is primarily due to the forces exercised by the rocking and gliding movements

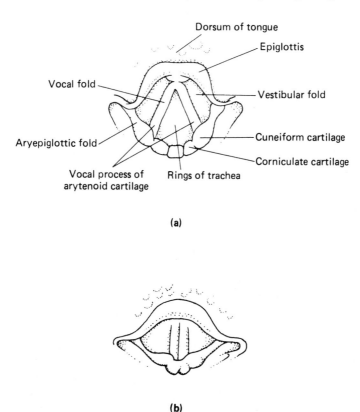

(a)

(b)

Fig. 21 View of larynx as seen with laryngoscope: (a) glottis open; (b) glottis closed

of the arytenoids. Just above the vocal cords is a second pair of folds, known as the *false vocal folds* (or *vestibular folds*), which seem to be uninvolved in speech.

The muscles of the larynx are divided into two types. *Extrinsic* muscles originate outside of the larynx and attach to the cartilages on the outside; their primary role is to move the larynx as a whole upwards and downwards—for example, in swallowing. *Intrinsic* muscles have their origins and endings within the larynx: their function is to move the arytenoid and cricoid cartilages, and to help in the process of contraction within the vocal cords. Two types of muscles in particular should be mentioned in this connection. One type causes the vocal cords to separate from the midline, or *abduct*—the *posterior cricoarytenoid* muscle. The other type causes the vocal cords to come together, or *adduct*—the *lateral cricoarytenoid*, and the two *arytenoid* (*oblique* and *transverse*) muscles. The muscle which forms the main part of the vocal cords themselves is known as the *vocalis* muscle. All intrinsic muscles of the larynx are supplied by branches of the vagus (Xth cranial) nerve. This nerve has two such branches: the *superior laryngeal nerve* supplies the cricothyroid muscle; the other intrinsic muscles are supplied by the *recurrent laryngeal nerves* ('recurrent', because the descending nerves pass below the level of the larynx and then loop upwards again—a feature which is especially noticeable on the left side, where the nerve takes a longer course (descending into the thorax and winding round the arch of the aorta), and where it is, accordingly, more vulnerable.

The question of how precisely the vocal cords operate, from a physiological viewpoint, has been the subject of controversy, and is still not wholly understood. The most widely-held theory maintains that the cords are set in vibration aerodynamically, solely by a reaction taking place between their elastic properties and the subglottal air pressure involved— the 'myoelastic' theory of voice production. An alternative theory, developed in the 1950s, argued that the cords are set in motion as a result of periodic neural stimulation and contraction of the muscles—the 'neurochronaxiac' theory.

The vocal cords have several functions. Their main role in speech is to vibrate in such a manner as to produce *voice*, a process known as *phonation*. When the cords are not vibrating, two main alternative positions are possible. They may be tightly closed, as when the breath is held—a process which upon release can produce a sound known as a *glottal stop* (as in a Cockney pronunciation of the middle consonant in *bottle* /'bɒʔl/). Or they may remain open, so that the breath flowing through the glottis produces audible friction, as in whispering, or the [h] sound. Other 'phonation types' are possible, by varying the mode of vibration of the vocal cords in various ways: for example, if the cords are made to vibrate very slowly, a 'creaky' voice quality is produced; a very fast, tense mode of vibration produces a 'falsetto' voice. Lastly, by varying the rate and strength of vibration of the vocal cords, changes in pitch and loudness can be introduced into speech.

Above the larynx, the air-stream is further modified by the shapes assumed by the vocal tract. Three main cavities are involved, and these act as the main *resonators* of the voice quality produced at the larynx: the *pharyngeal cavity*, the *oral cavity* and the *nasal cavity* (see Figure 22). The general term used in phonetics for the physiological movements involved in modifying the air-stream within these cavities is *articulation*. Sounds are classified in terms of their *place* and their *manner* of articulation within the vocal tract. Any specific part of the vocal tract involved in the production of a sound is called an *articulator*. Two kinds of articulators are distinguished: 'active' articulators are the movable parts of the vocal tract, such as the lips, tongue and lower jaw (or *mandible*); 'passive' articulators are those parts of the vocal tract which cannot move, but which provide the active articulators with points of reference, such as the upper teeth and the roof of the mouth. The whole range of articulators is illustrated in Figure 22. Two, the tongue and the soft palate, are of particular importance, from the point of view of speech pathology:

1 The tongue's importance lies in the fact that it is the organ of articulation most involved in the production of speech sounds—all the vowels, and the majority of the consonants (excluding only those made at the lips and in the throat). It consists of an extremely mobile muscle, covered with mucous membrane, or mucosa. It is divided into two areas: the anterior (oral) two-thirds is rough, being covered with tiny projections (*papillae*) which can rasp and hold food (it also contains the nerve-endings for taste); the posterior (pharyngeal) third is smooth, to facilitate swallowing. The blade of the tongue is loosely attached to the floor of the mouth by a vertical fold of mucous membrane, known as the *frenum* (or *frenulum*, i.e. a small frenum) of the tongue (which can be clearly seen when the tip of the tongue is raised and pulled back). The great mobility of the tongue is due to its sophisticated system of muscular control. The *extrinsic* muscles of the tongue, originating outside the tongue in the hyoid bone, mandible and skull, alter the position of the tongue in the mouth, and work, along with the *intrinsic* tongue muscles (i.e. those internal to the tongue), to change the tongue's shape. The intrinsic tongue muscle is unique in the body in that its fibres run in all three planes—vertical, lateral and horizontal fibres all interlacing with one another. Seven basic types of tongue movement are possible, using these muscles, permitting the tip, edges and centre of the tongue a fair degree of independent movement: a horizontal anterior-posterior movement of the body of the tongue, and of its tip/blade; a vertical superior/inferior movement of the body, and of the tip/blade; a transverse concave/convex movement; a spread/tapered contrast in the front part of the tongue; and a degree of central grooving. All of these movements are involved in the articulation of speech sounds, some sounds involving only two or three of these parameters (such as the vowels), other sounds involving far more (such as [s] or [ʃ]). The lateral view of the tongue in Fig. 22

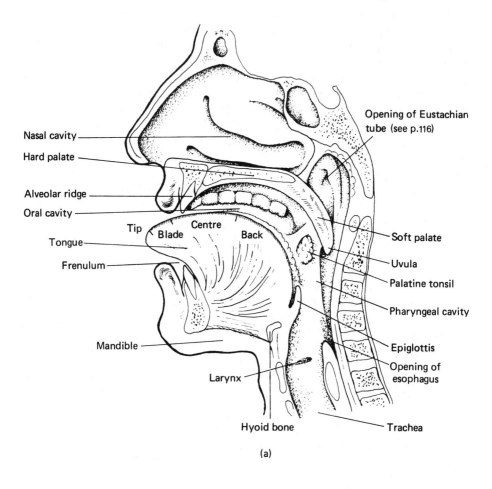

(a)

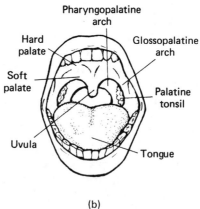

(b)

Fig. 22 (a) Sagittal section through the vocal tract (see p. 94); (b) frontal view of oral cavity

illustrates the main functional areas that are generally recognized (*tip*, *blade*, *centre* and *back*), but it obscures the median groove.

2 The soft palate (or *velum*, or *velo-pharyngeal sphincter*) is the mobile, muscular posterior extension of the hard palate (the immobile bony arch forming the roof of the mouth). It culminates in the uvula, a muscular flap easily visible when the mouth is wide open. Three muscular forces act on the soft palate, enabling it to be raised (largely through the *levator palatini* muscle), tensed (through the *tensor palatini* muscle) and lowered (though the *palatoglossus* and *palatopharyngeus* muscles). During normal respiration, the mouth is closed, and the soft palate is in its lowered position, air travelling in and out through the nose. For most of the sounds of speech, however, the soft palate is in its raised position, closing off the upper part of the pharynx, and thus enabling oral sounds to be produced. Poor control of the soft palate (see further, p. 175) may lead to audible nasal resonance and friction while producing oral sounds, and is a major cause of unintelligible or unacceptable speech.

The other active articulators in the vocal tract are, of course, important, but their effect is more localized. The lips are the next most important—a pair of fleshy folds used both for the expression of emotional feelings and for speech. The main muscle of the lips is the *orbicularis oris*, which both lips share, but there are several other muscular connections to other parts of the face, and it is these which enables the upper and the lower lips to have a considerable degree of independent movement (the lower lip being the more mobile). The configurations of the lips of importance for speech mainly involve degrees of lip-rounding and lip-spreading (as in the vowels) and degrees of tension in their contact (as in the production of various consonants). Less important is the mandible, as far as speech is concerned: the several muscles which control its raising/lowering, protrusion/retraction and lateral movement are more involved with such processes as chewing than with speech. And lastly, there is the active role of the pharynx in speech production: recent studies of the pharynx show it to be in constant movement during speech, but it is not clear what effects this movement has.

No reference has so far been made to the teeth. Few sounds are actually formed primarily using the teeth, but many consonants and vowels use the teeth as part of their articulatory basis, and it is remarkable how much misarticulation can be the result of any misalignment or deficiency in their number. The first teeth to grow are known as the *deciduous* teeth: these are 20 in number, 10 in each jaw. There are four *incisor* teeth (the flat, cutting teeth in the front of the mouth): one on either side of the dental midline (the *central* incisors), and one on either side of these (the *lateral* incisors). Next to the lateral incisors are the *canine* teeth, one on each side; and these are followed by the *molar* teeth, two on each side. Deciduous teeth in due course are replaced by 32 permanent teeth, 16 in each jaw (4 incisors, 2 canines, 4 *premolars*, and 6 molars—the most posterior pair on each side also being known as the *wisdom* teeth). The relationship between the teeth is seen in Figure 23. The normal alignment of the upper (maxillary) and lower (mandibular) jaw produces a complete pattern of contact between the teeth, known as *occlusion*. Various types of *malocclusion* occur, in which the misalignment of the teeth disallows this normal contact pattern (producing abnormal biting characteristics). There are also several types of teeth *malposition*, in relation to the jaw or to each other. Either of these abnormal conditions can affect articulation, sometimes severely, and are a major factor contributing to the unacceptability or unintelligibility of speech. The correction and prevention of such problems is the province of *orthodontics*.

So far, we have outlined speech sound production from the point of view of where in the vocal tract the modification to the air-stream takes place. On the basis of these distinctions, it is accordingly possible to classify sounds in terms of their place of articulation, and this is one of the main parameters recognized by phonetics (and usually represented horizontally on a sound

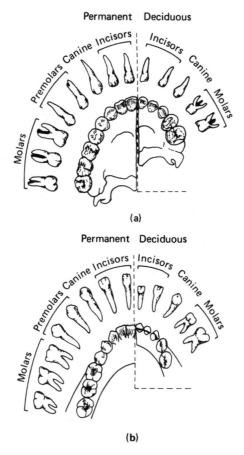

Fig. 23 Permanent and deciduous teeth of (a) upper and (b) lower jaw

classification chart, such as the one given in Fig. 24, which is that used by the International Phonetics Association, and known as the *International Phonetic Alphabet (IPA)*). This lateral view inevitably omits some of the place variations which can only be identified transversely, such as whether only one or both sides of the tongue is involved in an articulation; but it is valuable as far as it goes. The main consonantal divisions, according to place of articulation, can be read from front to back in the mouth (left to right) as follows (illustrations are from English, unless otherwise stated):

labial   both lips involved   [p] [b] [m]
labio-dental   lip against teeth   [f] [v]
dental   tongue against teeth   [θ] [ð]
alveolar   tongue against teeth-ridge   [t] [d]
palatal   tongue against hard palate   [ç] [j]
velar   tongue against velum   [k] [g]
uvular   tongue against uvula   [q] [G] (in Arabic)
pharyngeal   constriction in the pharynx   [ħ] [ʕ] (in Arabic)
glottal   constriction at glottis   glottal stop, whisper

Several other places can be recognized, between these. Vowels are all articulated in the area beneath the palatal-velar region, and are classified in terms of their relative position *front-central-back* and *high-mid-low*.

The vertical dimension of classification on the IPA chart handles the other type of factor which interferes with the air-stream in the vocal tract: manner of articulation. This refers to the *kind* of articulatory process used in a sound's production. The basic distinction between consonant and vowel is one of manner of articulation (the former involving a complete closure of the articulators, or a degree of narrowing which produces audible friction; the latter being more open). Several articulatory types are in fact recognized within the consonantal type, based on the type of closure made by the active articulators. If the closure is complete, the result is a *plosive* (as in [p], [b], [t]), *affricate* (as in [tʃ] and [dʒ]), or *nasal* (as in [m], [n]). If the closure is partial (along the centre of the mouth), the air is released around the sides of the closure, and the result is a *lateral* (as in [l]). If the closure is intermittent, the result is a *roll* (as in Scots [r]) or a *flap* (as in the [ɾ] of *very*). And if there is narrowing without complete closure, so that audible friction is produced, the result is a *fricative* (as in [f], [v], [s], [h]). Within vowels, classification is based on the number of auditory qualities distinguishable in the sound (*pure vowels*, such as [i] and [e]; *diphthongs*, such as [ei]), the position of the soft palate (whether *oral* or *nasal* vowels) and the type of lip position (whether *rounded* or *unrounded*). Some sounds are difficult to classify, sharing some of the properties of both vowels and consonants (the so-called *semi-vowels*, such as [w] and [ẏ], and the *frictionless continuants*, such as the r [ɹ] of *red*).

This classification is an adequate basis for analysing the sound *segments* of speech, but what about those features of speech which are not capable of being analysed into segments? These, the nonsegmental (or prosodic) aspects of speech have been referred to in Chapter 2 (p. 41). In terms of

	Bilabial	Labiodental	Dental, Alveolar, or Post-alveolar	Retroflex
Nasal	m	ɱ	n	ɳ
Plosive	p b		t d	ʈ ɖ
(Median) Fricative	φ β	f v	θ ð s z	ʂ ʐ
(Median) Approximant		ʋ	ɹ	ɻ
Lateral Fricative			ɬ ɮ	
Lateral (Approximant)			l	ɭ
Trill			r	
Tap or Flap			ɾ	ɽ
Ejective	p'		t'	
Implosive	ɓ		ɗ	
(Median) Click	ʘ		ʇ ʗ	
Lateral Click			ʖ	

(vertical labels: SONANTS (pulmonic air-stream mechanism); CONSONANTS (non-pulmonic air-stream))

DIACRITICS

- ₒ Voiceless n̥ d̥
- ᵥ Voiced s̬ t̬
- ʰ Aspirated tʰ
- ¨ Breathy-voiced b̤ a̤
- ₙ Dental t̪
- ₗ Labialized t̫
- ⌄ Palatalized t̬
- ~ Velarized or Pharyn-gealized ɫ, ɫ
- ₗ Syllabic n̩ l̩
- ˆ or ⌣ Simultaneous s͡f (but see also under the heading Affricates)

- ˙ or . Raised e˙, ẹ, ẹ w
- ˙ or ˌ Lowered e˙, ẹ, ẹ ʁ
- ₊ Advanced u+, u̟
- - or ˗ Retracted i̠, i˗, t̠
- ¨ Centralized ë
- ~ Nasalized ã
- ʳ, ˡ, ᴿ r-coloured aˡ
- : Long ɑ:
- · Half-long ɑ·
- ˘ Non-syllabic ŭ
- ˃ More rounded ɔ˃
- ˂ Less rounded y˂

OTHER SYMBOLS

- ɕ, ʑ Alveolo-palatal fricatives
- ʃ, ʒ Palatalized ʃ, ʒ
- ɼ Alveolar fricative trill
- ɺ Alveolar lateral flap
- ʄ Simultaneous ʃ and x
- ʃˢ Variety of ʃ resembling s, etc.
- ɪ = ι
- ʊ = ɷ
- ɜ = Variety of ə
- ɚ = r-coloured ə

Fig. 24 The International Phonetic Alphabet

Palato-alveolar	Palatal		Velar		Uvular		Labial-Palatal	Labial-Velar		Pharyngeal		Glottal	
		ɲ		ŋ	N								
	c	ɟ	k	g	q	ɢ		k͡p	g͡b			ʔ	
ʃ ʒ	ç	j	x	ɣ	χ	ʁ		ʍ		ħ	ʕ	h	ɦ
		j	ɰ				ɥ	w					
			ʌ										
					ʀ								
					ʀ								
		k'											
		ɠ											

Front		Back	VOWELS	Front		Back	
i	ɨ	ɯ	Close	y	ʉ	u	
ɪ				ʏ		ʊ	
e		ɤ	Half-close	ø		o	
	ə				ɵ		
ɛ		ʌ	Half-open	œ		ɔ	
æ	ɐ						
a		ɑ	Open	ɶ		ɒ	
Unrounded				Rounded			

STRESS, TONE (PITCH)

ˈ stress, placed at beginning of stressed syllable : ˌ secondary stress : ˉ high level pitch, high tone : ˍ low level : ´ high rising : ˏ low rising : ` high falling : ˎ low falling : ˆ rise-fall : ˇ fall-rise.

AFFRICATES can be written as digraphs, as ligatures, or with slur marks ; thus ts, tʃ, dʒ : ʦ tʃ ʤ : t͡s t͡ʃ d͡ʒ. c, ɟ may occasionally be used for tʃ, dʒ.

speech production, their origin is quite different from any of the other sounds so far described. The variables are primarily those of *pitch* (both pitch direction—the melody rising, falling, staying level etc.—and pitch range—the pitch level widening, narrowing etc.) and *loudness* (the different degrees of stress that can be given to the syllables of a word, or the overall loudness of a phrase or sentence). In addition, there are *tempo* variations, mainly noticeable through changes in the duration of segments, pauses, and in the overall speed and rhythm of an utterance. And lastly, there is a large group of 'tone of voice' effects usually referred to collectively under the heading of *timbre*. The best way of explaining what is involved in timbre is by way of a musical analogy: given an oboe and a clarinet, both playing the same note at the same loudness and for the same length of time, the perceived difference is one of timbre. In speech, timbre variations are the result of changes in muscular tension, resonance, and several other factors (see further, p. 173 ff.). The transcription of all these features is, as one might imagine, a much more difficult matter than with the phonetic segments above, and this aspect of phonetics has been relatively neglected in its application to speech pathology.[32]

Using this information about air-stream mechanisms, types of phonation and articulation, several types of speech pathology can be distinguished, and these are described in Chapter 4. These are often, though not always, associated with organic damage to the vocal organs, or to the muscles and nerves controlling them. The vocal organs are susceptible to any of the categories of disease outlined in Chapter 2 (pp. 21–2). Their medical investigation would proceed in a hospital ENT department, the relevant specialisms being: *otology*—the study of the ear and its diseases (see pp. 114 ff. below); *rhinology*—the study of the nose and its diseases; and *laryngology*—the study of the larynx and its diseases. It would be wrong to see the three areas involved as being independent of each other: diseases of the upper respiratory tract often spread to the ear (via the Eustachian tube—see Fig. 22); the nose and throat are often simultaneously affected by a single disease (as in the common cold); a nervous disease, such as facial nerve paralysis (in which the muscles of the face are weakened in varying degrees, as in Bell's palsy), may affect broad areas; there may be a *structural* abnormality affecting several parts of the vocal tract, as in cleft palate (see p. 187); and so on. But it is possible to make a classification of the main pathologies in regional terms, any of which could have an effect on the intelligibility or acceptability of speech.

Some of the common diseases affecting the nose and nasal cavity include colds, catarrh, the various types of *sinusitis* (inflammation of the air cavities, lined with mucous membrane, which communicate with the nose—the *paranasal sinuses*), nasal haemorrhage (*epistaxis*, or nose-bleeding) or the

---

[32] For an introduction to general phonetics, see J. D. O'Connor, *Phonetics* (Harmondsworth, Penguin 1973), P. Ladefoged, *A course in phonetics* (New York, Harcourt Brace 1975). A detailed study of speech physiology is W. J. Hardcastle, *Physiology of speech production* (London, Academic Press 1976).

introduction of foreign bodies into the nose, causing blockage and damage. There may be tumours[33] in the nasal cavity, which may grow until they interfere with respiratory and/or speech function. Likewise, polyps[34] may develop, with similar results. A common cause of an abnormal nasal voice is adenoids—a mass of lymphoid (gland-like) tissue on the posterior wall of the nasopharynx; it normally atrophies (reduces naturally in size) in children by 6–7 years, but it may hypertrophy (increase in size, independent of the natural growth of the body), and need to be surgically removed. A similar development may affect the *tonsils*, found on the lateral walls of the pharynx below the soft palate, and visible on either side at the back of the mouth (see Fig. 22). Lastly, we should note the (rare) possibility of congenital malformation of the nasal cavity, which in its extreme form may consist of a complete blocking (*atresia*) of the posterior openings (*nares*, pron. /ˈnɛəriːz/, singular *naris*) of the nose. The specific name of the posterior nares is the *choanae* (singular *choana*, pron. /kəʊˈeɪnə/, and the condition is thus called *choanal atresia*.

A very wide range of disorders may affect the throat. One of the commonest is the *acute laryngitis* and *pharyngitis* which arises from infection in the upper respiratory tract. The larynx may also be frequently affected by trauma—wounds, blows to the neck, foreign bodies etc. Various kinds of lesion may affect the vocal cords. *Nodules*, or *nodes*, may develop as a result of misuse of the vocal cords (see further, p. 177), as may *ulcers* ('contact ulcers'). Polyps may form, as also may firmer, more fibrous tumours (*fibromas*), and tiny wart-like swellings known as *papillomata* (singular *papilloma*, pron. /pæpɪˈləʊmə/). Some of these conditions are illustrated in Figure 25.

These are all benign lesions. Malignant neoplasms affecting the throat, and the vocal cords in particular (*carcinoma*—cancer—*of the larynx*) can be treated with radiotherapy, and if this fails, with surgical removal of the larynx (*laryngectomy*). After such removal, the trachea cannot be rejoined to the pharynx, as the protective function of the larynx is lost, and food would spill uncontrollably into the lungs. The defect in the pharynx is therefore closed during the operation (see Fig. 26), and the trachea opens directly onto the neck—a *tracheostomy*. (A tracheostomy may also be made as a simple opening into the trachea without disturbing the larynx, in a patient who has a serious respiratory blockage or insufficiency). In such patients (*laryngectomees*), a wholly new way of producing speech must be learned (see further, p. 175). Nervous disease may also affect the vocal cords, specifically the paralysis of the laryngeal nerves (*recurrent laryngeal nerve palsy*): this usually affects the left nerve, causing immobility of the cord on

---

[33] A tumour is a new growth of cells or tissues which develops independently of the rest of the body. A *malignant* tumour is one which destroys surrounding tissues, and can extend into a surrounding area often at some distance from the original site (a process known as *metastasis*). A *benign* tumour does not act in this way.

[34] A polyp, once developed, is a smooth, spherical projection composed of neoplastic tissue (cf. p. 22); it may have a broad base (*sessile polyp*) or a narrow base (*pedunculated polyp*), mushroom-like in shape.

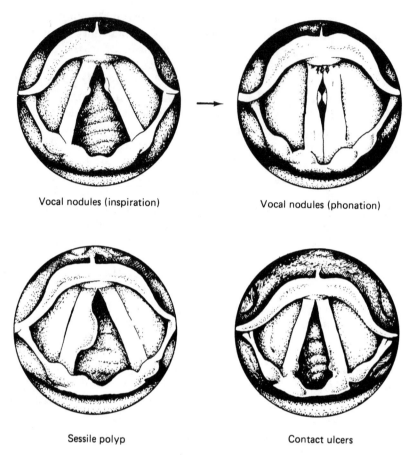

Vocal nodules (inspiration)   Vocal nodules (phonation)

Sessile polyp   Contact ulcers

Fig. 25 Some abnormal laryngeal conditions

that side. There are some rare congenital disorders affecting the larynx—partial or complete atresia of the glottis (*congenital vocal web*). And lastly, there are the results on the larynx of the normal process of degeneration in old age—such as the stiffening of the laryngeal joints that accompanies arthritis. All of these conditions will affect speech in some way: their effects are discussed further in Chapter 4 (p. 177).[35]

Step 4 Acoustic transmission

The study of the physical transmission of sound is known as *acoustics*. In this chapter, we shall be concerned only with speech sounds, and their transmission through the medium of air. From the point of view of speech

[35] Laryngeal disease is discussed in T. Bull and J. Cook, *Speech therapy and ENT surgery* (Oxford, Blackwell 1976), E. H. Miles Foxen, *Lecture notes on diseases of the ear, nose and throat* (Oxford, Blackwell, 4th edn, 1976), Chs. 16ff.

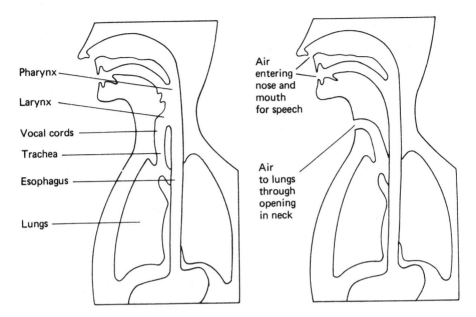

Fig. 26 (a) before and (b) after laryngectomy

pathology, the main relevance of this subject is its role in providing an alternative description of speech sounds to that provided by articulatory phonetics, which can then be used in techniques of assessment and remediation. It is, after all, extremely difficult to describe what sounds are like from the viewpoint of the listener: how would you describe the auditory effect on you of an [l] sound, or a [v]? All kinds of impressionistic labels have been used to try to pin down these auditory qualities, but they are extremely elusive. Words such as 'dark', 'hissy', 'sharp' (and several thousand others) can be used; but the trouble is that different people use these labels in different ways. Is there a difference between a voice that might be said to be 'hoarse', 'harsh', husky', 'rasping' . . .? Some people use these terms as synonyms; others give them subtly different senses. This is a major problem for the speech pathologist, as we shall see (p. 176). It is therefore extremely useful to have available an objective set of reference points for speech, so that sounds can be identified and discussed without the distortion imposed by differences in our hearing response and cultural backgrounds. And this is what acoustics provides.

Any source of vibration will initiate movement in the air particles which are adjacent to it. The air particles are displaced around their position of rest, travelling backwards and forwards in a movement known as *oscillation*. The air particles do not permanently leave their positions, but oscillate around it, each particle transmitting its vibratory movement to the next, in much the same way as waves are set up in water. Two characteristics of this oscillatory movement are fundamental. The number of times the particle oscillates in a given timespan (usually a second) is known as its *frequency*. The maximum extent of its oscillation is known as its *amplitude*. The relation between these two variables is shown in Fig. 27. The whole of the movement from A to B to C and back again to A is known as a *cycle*. Frequency of a sound is thus measured in 'cycles per second', these days summarized under the label Hertz (Hz) (after the German physicist, Heinrich Rudolf Hertz (1857–94), who first broadcast and received radio waves). We can hear sounds whose frequency is within the range of 20 Hz–20,000 Hz. The amplitude of a sound is determined partly by the energy which produced the sound in the first place, and partly by what happens to the sound as it is transmitted through the air. As its energy dies, so its oscillations become weaker (they 'decay', or are *damped*). The sound's amplitude may also be aided, if its vibratory movement causes objects in its path to vibrate in sympathy with it (*resonate*). Depending on the size, shape and texture of the object, it will have a *resonating frequency*, i.e. a 'favourite' frequency at which the maximum vibratory response will be obtained to a sound which reaches it. A buzzing sound in a room, for example, may start some objects vibrating loudly and not others: these objects thus have the resonating frequency of the buzz. From this point of view, the vocal tract can be seen as a resonating tube. The sound produced at the larynx, as we have seen, is modified in various ways by the organs of articulation. Put in acoustic terms, these organs have been made to vibrate as a consequence of the airstream passing them. By altering their shapes, we alter their resonating characteristics, and thus the quality of the sound.

The simple wave illustrated below in Fig. 27 is the sort of 'pure' wave-form (a *sinusoidal* wave) that would be produced by an object such as a tuning-fork. The wave-forms of speech are much more complex than this,

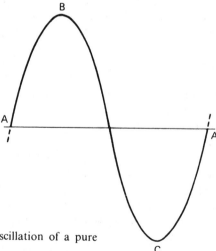

Fig. 27 One cycle of oscillation of a pure sound-wave

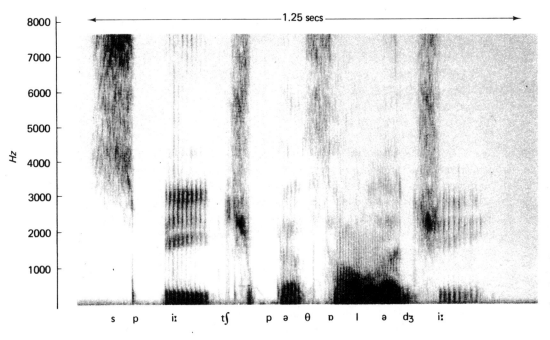

Fig. 28 Spectrogram of the phrase *speech pathology*

containing many components as a result of the several vibratory sources in the vocal tract. The complete set of frequency components in a sound wave is known as its *spectrum*. The analysis and measurement of speech-sound spectra is the province of acoustic phonetics. Some sounds such as [s] and [ʃ] are largely composed of high frequency components; others, such as the vowels, are largely composed of lower frequencies. One way of seeing these frequencies is by using a *spectrograph*, a device which analyses sounds into their component frequencies and prints these as a series of lines on specially sensitized paper. A typical *spectrogram* is given in Fig. 28. The time-scale of my articulation of *speech pathology* is from left to right—1·25 secs in all. The frequencies of the sound go from bottom to top, and are given on the left side of the spectrogram, in Hz, from 0 to 8000 (frequencies above this cannot be represented on this type of display, but these first 8000 contain most of the information needed to understand the physics of speech). The varying strength, or amplitude, of the different frequencies is represented by the varying degree of blackness of the striations on the spectrogram. Thus for the vowel [iː] in this spectrogram, three of the places where the acoustic energy is most concentrated (three of the *formants*) are around 280 Hz (the vowels 'first formant'), 1900 Hz (the 'second formant') and 2900 Hz (the 'third formant'). All sounds can be acoustically characterized in this way, either by specifying their formants (as with the vowels, and with certain consonants) or by identifying other acoustic characteristics (such as the random noise in the upper part of the chart, characteristic of [s], or the bend (*transition*) in the formants for [iː], showing the influence of the preceding [p] sound).

The other main technique of measuring the characteristics of sound is in terms of its intensity. The unit involved is the *decibel* (dB). The mathematical derivation of this unit is complex, requiring that we take into account several related concepts. We begin with the basic concept of *energy*, or power, which can be measured in various ways (by such units as watts, or horsepower). The result of energy is *pressure* being exercised against some object; this, too, can be measured, in terms of the amount of force being applied to a unit area of surface. *Bars* (millibars etc.) are a well-known way of measuring large-scale pressure variations on weather charts. For small-scale variations in pressure, the unit involved is known as the *dyne*.[36] A zero reference point for the measurement of differences in intensity has been established, of ·0002 dynes per cm² (roughly equal to the smallest audible pressure increase). The intensity of a sound, relative to this reference point, is known as its *sound pressure level*, or *SPL*, and it is this which is measured in decibels.[37] Because of the enormous range of SPLs possible, the decibel scale has been made logarithmic, which makes it much easier to work with: this means, for example, that a sound which has been estimated as having a SPL of 20 dB is not just twice as intense as one of 10 dB—it is 100 times (10×10) as intense; similarly, 30 dB is 1000 times ($10 \times 10 \times 10$) as intense; and so on. The numbers get very large, it is evident, but this only reflects the reality of our sophisticated hearing mechanism. The strongest sounds that we can hear without pain are some 10 million million times stronger than the minimally audible sound referred to above. Some typical decibel levels for everyday objects are:

0 dB	sound is just distinguishable from silence
20 dB	whispering at about a metre distance
60 dB	conversation at about a metre distance
100 dB	a pneumatic drill at about 5 metres distance
120 dB	jet aircraft overhead
140 dB	jet aircraft at a few metres distance

Based upon the combined scales of frequency and intensity, a graph of hearing ability has been constructed, known as an *audiogram*. An example of an audiogram form is given in Figure 29. The frequency range of the sounds is given across the top of the form from left to right. Decibel loss is indicated vertically: the top of the scale is normal, and the degree of loss is indicated at 10 dB increments as one moves downwards. Thus, for example, a sound might be presented to a patient at 500 Hz, and the intensity of this sound gradually lessened until finally it would be below the threshold of that

[36] The relation between bars and dynes is that one bar = 1 million dynes per cm².
[37] The underlying unit is known as a *bel* (after Alexander Graham Bell (1847–1922)). The decibel is one tenth of a bel; it is used because of its greater convenience in handling the small variations involved.

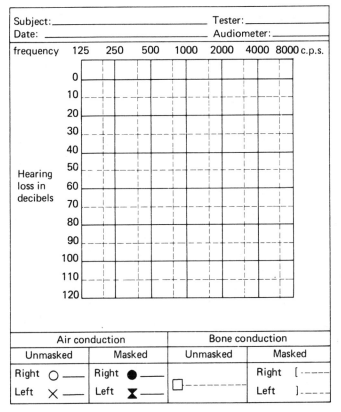

Fig. 29 A typical audiogram form

person's hearing. A theoretical normal hearing response would be a straight line at 0 on the audiogram; in practice, a certain amount of fluctuation around this line is generally encountered in normal subjects. The further away from this line the response pattern is, the more it will be considered abnormal: several such patterns are illustrated later in this book (see p. 138 and 139). The audiogram records only responses to artificially-generated pure tones, as produced by an audiometer, and not to the complex tones of speech. The audiologist marks on the audiogram the hearing thresholds of the person being tested, i.e. the lowest-intensity levels capable of giving him an awareness of sensation. Separate thresholds may be recorded for sound perceived through the air and through bone (see further, p. 131). Standard symbols for air conduction are 0 for the right ear and X for the left. Bone conduction symbols in British use are] for right ear response and [for left.[38]

[38] There is no international agreement concerning the symbols for bone conduction: some texts use the opposite convention to that described above; another system uses > and < for unmasked and ▷ and ◁ for masked bone-conduction responses (right and left respectively). △ and □ are sometimes used for masked air-conduction responses.

One other point concerning the acoustic analysis of speech should be made, as it is a regular source of confusion, and that is to distinguish the terminology we use when describing the physical characteristics of speech from that used when describing speech in auditory terms. So far, in this section, the description has been physical: sounds have been described in terms of their physical *dimensions*, of frequency, intensity (or amplitude) and time. Our *perception* of these variables is an altogether different matter, and is described in terms of sensory *attributes*, of *pitch*, *loudness* and *duration*. Pitch, for example, is our perception of sounds in terms of how high or low they are. It is largely, but by no means exclusively, associated with variations in frequency. To increase the frequency of a sound will generally result in our perceiving the sound as being higher in pitch; but there is no easy one-to-one correlation between these two notions. Experiments have shown that if we increase the intensity or duration of a sound, while holding the frequency steady, our judgements of pitch are affected. And a similar complexity exists for the other variables. When we have been talking of decibels, audiograms, and so on, therefore, we have been talking about some of the physical characteristics of sound, which we use as a means (the only practicable means we have) of investigating people's ability to hear (i.e. their perception of pitch and loudness). When we try to measure pitch and loudness, as perceptual responses, directly, different scales are involved (pitch being measured in units known as *mels*, loudness in units known as *sones*). There is no one-to-one relationship between these scales, and the physical scales used above. Their investigation falls within the study of auditory perception (see p. 119)—part of the final step in the communication chain.[39]

Step 5 Auditory reception

The first step in the reception component of the communication chain is when sound is received by the ear. To understand the process, the ear is usually studied under three headings, corresponding to the main anatomical/physiological structures involved: the outer ear, the middle ear, and the inner ear (see Figure 30).

The outer ear
This consists of the visible part of the ear (the *auricle*, or *pinna*) and the narrow passage which leads to the eardrum, known as the *external auditory canal* (or *external auditory meatus* (pron. /miːˈeɪtəs/, a term meaning an end-stopped passage). The pinna is a nonmobile structure, consisting primarily of cartilage, formed from six rounded prominences, or tubercles. It has some function as an area for erogenous stimulation, but as far as language is concerned, its role seems minor, being mainly involved in the focusing of sound waves into the ear, and assisting the process of sound localization (i.e.

[39] On the acoustics of speech, see P. B. Denes and E. N. Pinson, *The speech chain* (New York, Anchor Books 1973), esp. Chs. 3, 7, D. B. Fry (ed.), *Acoustic phonetics* (Cambridge, CUP 1976).

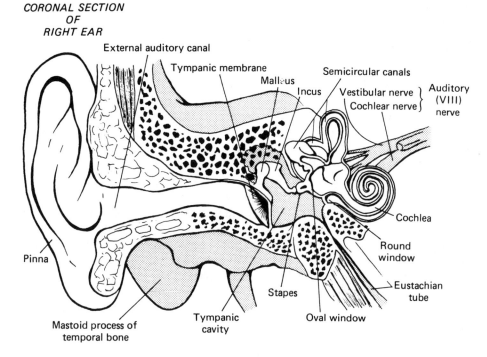

CORONAL SECTION
OF
RIGHT EAR

Fig. 30 The structure of the ear

our ability to detect where a sound is coming from). The external auditory canal is about 2·5 cm long, and ends at the eardrum. Its outer part contains hairs and glands which secrete wax (*cerumen*). The canal acts as a small amplifier for certain sound frequencies (between 3000 and 4000 Hz), thus making weak sounds at these frequencies much more perceptible than they would otherwise be. The presence of the canal also helps to protect the sensitive eardrum to some extent from changes in temperature and humidity—and also from physical damage (though the ingenuity with which small children can insert implements right inside their ears is well attested!).

The middle ear
The eardrum, or *tympanic membrane*, separates the outer ear from the middle ear. It lies at an angle of about 55° across the whole of the canal; it is thus roughly circular in shape, and joined firmly to the walls of the canal. It consists primarily of a fibrous tissue with important elastic properties, enabling it to vibrate when sound waves reach it. The shape and tension of the tympanic membrane cause the vibrations to be focused at a prominence (or *umbo*) near its centre, and thus transferred to the first of the bones of the middle ear, which is firmly attached to the membrane.

The middle ear chamber is a cavity (the *tympanic cavity*) in the bones of the skull, about 15 mm long and 15 mm high. The cavity is filled with air, because there is a direct connection to the nose and throat via the Eustachian tube (after the Italian anatomist, G. E. Eustachio (1520–74)), which enters the middle ear at its anterior end. The tube is normally closed, but such activities as yawning or swallowing open it (often making a clicking sound in the ear). The need for this opening is to maintain the pressure level of the middle ear with that on the other side of the eardrum. If the pressure outside were greater than that inside, the eardrum would become deformed and function less efficiently. By allowing air into the middle ear, this possibility is lessened.

The primary function of the middle ear is to turn the sound vibrations which reach the eardrum into mechanical movement—movement which will then be transmitted to the inner ear. It does this by using a system of three tiny bones, known as the auditory *ossicles*. These bones are the smallest in the body; they are suspended from the walls of the tympanic cavity by ligaments, and are delicately hinged together, so that vibrations can be passed smoothly between them. The three bones have been given their names because of their physical resemblance to items from the blacksmith's forge. The most lateral ossicle is the *malleus*, or hammer: this is attached to the inner side of the eardrum by its handle, from whence it picks up sound vibrations. These are then transmitted to the *incus*, or anvil, which in turn joins with the head of the third ossicle, the *stapes*, or stirrup. The base, or *footplate*, of the stapes fits into an opening in the bony wall which forms the boundary between middle and inner ear: this opening, known as the *oval window*, is the means of transferring the vibrations into the fluid-filled inner ear.

This system of bony connections may seem a complicated way of getting vibrations from point A to point B, but it has several advantages. Chief amongst these is that the process acts as a kind of leverage system, which enables these vibrations to be greatly amplified (by a factor of about 35) by the time they reach the inner ear. As the inner ear is filled with fluid (see below), vibrations would very readily get lost, without this amplification; the system thus allows the inner ear to pick up more sound than would otherwise be possible. A second function of the bony network of the middle ear is that it helps to protect the inner ear from sudden, very loud sounds. The muscles which control the movement of the eardrum and the stapes function in such a way that they lessen the chances of massive vibrations hitting the inner ear and causing damage. Unfortunately, the time it takes for these muscles to come into operation is not so rapid that the inner ear can be protected from all such sounds; and in fact damage to the eardrum or the inner ear does occur.

The inner ear
This is a system of small interconnecting cavities and passageways within the bones of the skull, sometimes referred to as the *labyrinth*, or *aural labyrinth*. The system has two main parts. The *semicircular canals* (or *vestibular canals*)

are a series of passages organized into three loops set at angles to each other (anterior, posterior and lateral). The canals control our sense of balance. They are filled with fluid, and contain many tiny hairs, attached to nerve-endings: the movement of the head and body causes the fluid to move in the canal; this moves the hairs and causes impulses in the associated nerves. The other main part of the inner ear, and the part with which we are primarily concerned, is the *cochlea*, a cavity which is coiled, resembling a snail's shell. It is about 35 mm in length, and coils 2¾ times. The primary function of the cochlea is to turn the mechanical vibrations produced by the middle ear into nerve impulses, capable of being transmitted to the brain.

The cochlea is divided along most of its length into an upper chamber (the *scala vestibuli*) and a lower chamber (the *scala tympani*) (see Fig. 31). Separating these chambers is the *cochlear duct*, which has a complex internal structure of its own (see below). Both chambers are filled with a clear, viscous (i.e. sticky, slow-moving) fluid known as *perilymph*. Vibrations enter this fluid in the scala vestibuli from the middle ear, via the oval window (cf. above); they are then transmitted all the way around the cochlea, passing from upper to lower chamber through an opening in the cochlear partition at the end, or *apex* of the cochlea (the *helicotrema*), and finishing at a second opening in the wall of the middle ear, sealed with a membrane, called the *round window*. This permits fluid vibrations to travel freely in the perilymph, the round window yielding outwards when the footplate in the oval window moves inward, and vice versa (since perilymph, like all fluids, is incompressible).

The *cochlear duct* is separated from the upper and lower chambers of the

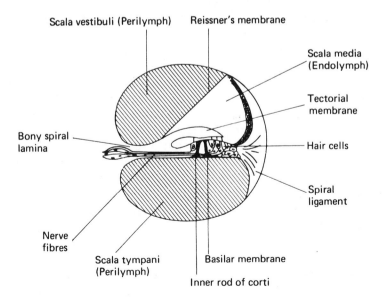

Fig. 31 Cross-sectional view of the cochlea

cochlea by membranes, and filled with a potassium-rich clear fluid, known as *endolymph*. The membrane which separates the cochlear duct from the scala vestibuli is known as *Reissner's membrane* (after the German anatomist, E. Reissner (1824–78)); the membrane which separates the duct from the scala tympani is known as the *basilar membrane*. One end of the basilar membrane is attached to a bony process, or shelf; the other to a ligament (the *spiral ligament*) on the outside wall of the cochlea. This membrane is very narrow at the cochlea's basal end (about ·04 mm) and gradually becomes thicker as it approaches the apical end (where it is about 0·5 mm). The importance of this is that the basilar membrane is thus able to respond differentially to different vibratory pressures: high frequencies of vibration primarily affect its narrow end; certain lower frequencies the thicker end; and other low frequencies activate the entire membrane.[40] An analogy is often drawn here with the strings of a piano: the thin, taut strings respond best to high frequencies, whereas the heavy and looser strings respond best to low frequencies. Indeed, the uncoiled basilar membrane has been compared to a kind of piano keyboard—though the analogy is not a particularly good one, and enormously underestimates the complex characteristics of this system's properties in responding to sound.

Resting on the basilar membrane is the highly sensitive organ of hearing, called the *organ of Corti* (discovered by the Italian anatomist, Alfonso Corti (1822–76) in 1836). Its task is to translate the mechanical movements of the membrane into nerve impulses. It contains a systematic arrangement of cells covered with very fine hairs, distributed in rows and layers along the membrane: these *hair cells* act as sensory receptors, picking up the pressure movements in the endolymph. The cells synapse with fibres from the VIIIth cranial (auditory) nerve; their movement is turned electrochemically into nerve impulses along this nerve, and thus are sent to the brain.

Anything which interferes with the normal structure and function of the ear is likely to promote a degree of hearing loss. The outer ear may be affected, e.g. if it contains abnormal amounts of wax, is penetrated by foreign bodies, or is inflamed as the result of infection (*otitis externa*). The tympanic membrane can be damaged, and perhaps ruptured ('perforated'), by trauma such as a foreign body, a blow, or an explosion. The majority of ear complaints, however, affect the middle ear. Particularly common is acute bacterial inflammation of the middle ear (*acute otitis media*), the infection having travelled into the ear along the Eustachian tube from the upper respiratory tract. If the infection persists (*chronic otitis media*) the risk of damage is much increased, and surgical intervention may be necessary. Obstruction to the Eustachian tube (e.g. by overgrown adenoids) may lead to an infection causing the middle ear to be filled with fluid; this fluid becomes increasingly viscous, and results in the condition of *secretory otitis*

[40] This is the so-called 'place' theory of pitch perception. There is also a 'frequency' or 'temporal' theory of pitch perception, in which the cochlea is viewed rather like a microphone, transmitting impulses to the auditory nerve; pitch is then determined by the frequency of the impulses along the nerve.

media (popularly known as 'glue ear'). To drain the ear, a tube can be inserted through the tympanic membrane (in a procedure known as *myringotomy*). *Otosclerosis* is a further common problem affecting the middle ear; it refers to a condition where new bone develops in the region of the base (or footplate) of the stapes, markedly reducing its mobility and thus its ability to transmit vibrations to the inner ear. In the operation of *stapedectomy*, the stapes is removed and replaced by a prosthesis (i.e. an artificial substitute), in the form of a small piston which is placed so as to join the incus to the oval window.

The inner ear, and particularly the cochlea, is very susceptible to damage, from a variety of sources. Diseases such as rubella (German measles), mumps and meningitis can have a direct effect on the cochlea, as can the excessive use of certain drugs (such as aspirin). The efficiency of the cochlea may also deteriorate if the ear is exposed to very loud noises over long periods (as in some factories and some discos); and there are in fact laws governing the ear protection of workers in noisy conditions (though not yet in discos!). There are also some congenital malformations which affect the inner ear. In none of these cases is it possible to repair the damage done to the inner ear. Too little is known about this structure for clear procedures to have developed. One recent line of research has been into *cochlear implanting*. Cochlear implants are tiny wires, implanted in the cochlea, which pick up signals from a transmitter placed within a hearing aid. They can produce a sensation of sound, but it takes a while for a patient to learn how to decode the sound he hears, as the effects this technique produces are some remove away from the normal. As a technique, also, it is used only for those patients who are profoundly deaf, as the operation is a *complete* substitute for normal hearing.

The branch of medicine which deals with diseases of the ear is known as *otology*; the specialist is an *otologist*. His role, and that of the audiologist, is discussed further in the section on deafness in Chapter 4.[41]

Step 6 Neurological transmission and brain decoding

Ironically, this has to be the shortest section of this chapter, though its importance to the communication chain is obviously crucial. The unfortunate fact of the matter is that the processes which affect nerve impulses along the VIII nerve en route to the brain are little understood. The various steps in the transmission process are fairly well established, from an anatomical and physiological point of view, but from a psychoacoustic angle much less is known. *Psychoacoustics* studies the way in which the brain responds to sound, and investigates the nature of our sensations when we listen to auditory stimuli (*auditory perception*). It must be stressed that the

[41] Further reading: P. B. Denes and E. N. Pinson, *The speech chain* (New York, Anchor Books 1973), Ch. 5; J. L. Northern and M. P. Downs, *Hearing in children* (Baltimore, Williams & Wilkins 1978), esp. Chs. 2, 3; E. H. Miles Foxen, *Lecture notes on diseases of the ear, nose and throat* (Oxford, Blackwell, 4th edn, 1976), Chs. 1–15.

psychoacoustic answer to the question 'What do we hear?' is very different from the articulatory and physical answers provided above. Two people may both be presented with the same sound, but 'hear' it in very different ways—as can be demonstrated by getting subjects to react to known sound stimuli, and observing the differences in their behaviour (e.g. whether they judge two sounds as being the same in pitch, loudness or duration).

A brief reference to some of the factors involved in auditory perception will illustrate the complexity of what is involved. Perception studies deal with the way an organism detects, discriminates, interprets and reacts to a stimulus. As soon as it is phrased like this, the great ambiguity of the term 'hearing' presents itself. When we say we have 'heard' a sound, what do we mean? At least these three aspects must be considered:

1 Has there been any automatic reaction to the sound stimulus? For example, newborn infants display a range of automatic reflex responses to sounds, including the twitching of the eyelid (at certain intensities) and the contraction/dilation of the pupils (at certain frequencies)—known as the *cochleopalpebral* and *cochleopupillary* reflexes, respectively. There is also a general acoustic muscle reflex, which causes variations in respiration and heart beat—one of the main ways in which research can be carried out into the developing sense of speech sound in the infant.

2 Has the sound stimulus been consciously detected? For a sound to be detected, there needs to be a certain minimum of stimulation provided (the *absolute threshold* of the stimulus).

3 Once a sound has been detected, we need to be able to recognize repeated instances of the stimulus as being the same (*recognition*) and to identify when other stimuli are different (*discrimination*). How different do two stimuli have to be in order for the brain to be able to perceive that they are different? The minimum difference in magnitude is known as the *difference threshold*. The abbreviation 'JND' is often used, when the auditory psychologist is talking about the difference between stimuli: 'just noticeable difference'. Myelination seems to be a crucial factor in the nervous system's ability to discriminate stimuli (cf. p. 74).

These thresholds are affected by several factors. For example, there is the phenomenon of sensory *adaptation*: if a stimulus is repeatedly presented, we become less sensitive to its presence, and finally come to ignore it altogether. Sounds that are regularly a part of our environment we ignore—unless something happens which draws our attention to them (cf. below). Fatigue is another factor which affects our auditory *acuity* (i.e. the sharpness with which we are able to detect and discriminate sound). The presence of *masking* sounds in the environment will be a factor, i.e. noise which interferes with the audibility of another sound. The controlled use of masking is in fact one way in which audiologists can establish the different roles and abilities of the two ears (see the audiogram in Fig. 29): a noise is played to one ear while the opposite ear is being tested.

Any of the above factors will play an important part in a discussion of hearing; but there is one further factor which has not so far been mentioned, and its influence too is crucial. This is the notion of *auditory attention*. Attention refers to the brain's ability to focus on certain aspects of a complex perceptual experience, and to ignore others. Attention can therefore be *selective*, and a great deal of research has gone on into the factors which control this selectivity. We are evidently able to exercise a great deal of control over our attention—as is illustrated by the 'cocktail-party' phenomenon, in which we are able to attend selectively to any one out of a series of simultaneously-occurring conversations going on around us. One major factor is semantic relevance: for instance, if someone mentions our name within the hubbub of the cocktail party, our attention is focused in that direction. Putting this in another way, what has happened is that we have begun to 'hear attentively'—or in other words, to *listen*. It is for this reason that listening is distinguished from hearing, in discussion of this subject. And it is listening which is prerequisite for the more complex processes of linguistic interpretation and response.[42]

---

[42] See further P. B. Denes and E. N. Pinson, *The speech chain* (New York, Anchor Books 1973), Chs. 6, 8; E. R. Hilgard, R. C. Atkinson and R. L. Atkinson, *Introduction to psychology* (New York, Harcourt Brace Jovanovich, 5th edn. 1971), Chs. 5, 6; B. Moore, *Introduction to the psychology of hearing* (London, Macmillan 1977); on speech perception in particular, H. H. Clark and E. V. Clark, *Psychology and language* (New York, Harcourt Brace Jovanovich 1977), Ch. 5.

4

The classification of linguistic pathologies

Earlier chapters have described the main variables which need to be taken into account when commencing the investigation of linguistic disability. We can now use this information, and specifically the framework provided by the communication chain, to help construct a classificatory system, in which the different kinds of abnormal language behaviour can be incorporated. But where to start? There can, it seems, be breakdowns at any point along the communication chain. Which category of problem should we address first? With those linguistic problems that result from neurological causes? or from auditory causes? or, more generally, does it matter whether we deal first with disabilities on the production side of the chain, or on the reception side?

Where we start will depend on our purpose. If we are investigating the development of disability chronologically, starting with the infant, then it will make sense to begin with the reception side, for some kind of input is obviously prerequisite if language is to develop. On the other hand, if our concern were primarily to differentially diagnose a series of adult patients on the basis of their language use, then a sensible way to proceed would be on the basis of their production patterns. In short, there is no single, best way of working through the steps of the communication chain. The organization of the later part of this chapter is, to a considerable extent, arbitrary.

Before we proceed to a description of the various pathologies, however, it is useful to consider some of the general principles guiding our approach. The main aim is to classify abnormal linguistic behaviour into categories that make medical and behavioural sense. But this is not a straightforward task. Several attempts have been made to define two or three very broad types of pathology, as a preliminary to more detailed investigation, and several of these initial classifications have been influential in shaping the present-day conception of the field. None of them are without criticism, however.

Production disorders v. reception disorders

This classification would seem to follow on nicely from the communication chain model presented in Chapter 3, and indeed it is helpful to some extent.

It coincides with the division between motor and sensory, and it does have clinical (especially therapeutic) relevance. But it should be plain, following our discussion of feedback (p. 58), that such a classification is very much an oversimplification. A purely auditory deficit can, and invariably does, lead to major problems of production, as we shall see in our discussion of deafness (p. 129). A purely production problem, such as stuttering, can raise difficulties of listening and comprehension (see p. 169). And when we deal with disorders of the central nervous system, such as aphasia, or the psychopathological syndromes, it proves extremely difficult to disentangle the two. It is commonplace to talk of 'expressive' (i.e. production) and 'receptive' aphasics, as we shall see (p. 142); but the majority of aphasic patients have problems that stem from both motor and sensory causes. Likewise, in children who have failed to develop language normally (see p. 160), the issue of whether there is primarily a production or reception problem in the brain may be unresolvable. The distinction between disorders of production and disorders of reception, then, is best seen as a means of guiding, but never of constraining, research and classification.

Organic disorders v. functional disorders

This distinction is also commonly encountered in language pathology. It is a consequence of the priority given to the medical model of analysis (cf. Chapter 2), whereby disorders are divided into two broad types: those where there is a clear organic (anatomical, physiological, neurological) cause and those where there is not. Various terms are used to refer to the latter category (e.g. psychogenic, psychological), but the most widespread term is 'functional'. So, for example, if a person loses the ability to make his vocal cords vibrate, and there is plainly a neurological cause for this, the voice disorder would be classified as organic (see further, p. 177). On the other hand, if an ENT examination could establish no cause, it would be concluded that there were probably psychological reasons for the problem, and the diagnosis would be functional. Other disorders, for example in articulation and fluency, can also be classified in this way. However, the apparently clearcut nature of this division is misleading—as we have already seen in Chapter 2 (p. 25), where a case-study was reported of someone whose problems seemed due to a combination of organic and psychological factors. And this is so often the case: either it is plain that both types of factor are involved (as with many voice disorders) or it is unclear which of the two types are involved (as with depressive illnesses, cf. p. 69). There are also cases where the expected straightforward correlations do not obtain—for example, cases of clear organic damage, where the patient has somehow managed to *compensate*, by using other parts of his vocal apparatus, and produces clear or reasonable speech. There are plainly many degrees of affectedness under either heading—degrees of organic damage interacting with degrees of functional lack of control—and in such a circumstance, the need for care in using the distinction should be obvious.[1]

Speech disorders v. language disorders

This classical distinction is still in widespread use, though with the development of recent work in linguistics its applicability is increasingly being questioned. The origins of the distinction lie in the difference between 'symbolic' and 'nonsymbolic' aspects of communication. Certain aspects of communication have as their primary role the communication of meaning: they have a symbolic function. By contrast, other aspects of communication have no direct involvement with meaning; their presence is an incidental result of the choice of communicative medium; they do not affect the meaning at all (are 'nonsymbolic'). Grammar and vocabulary were considered to be the main symbolic factors in communication; and when speech was the medium of communication involved, it was the phonetic characteristics of speech which were considered to be nonsymbolic. The former factors were grouped under the heading of *language*; the latter were grouped under the heading of speech. The position can be represented as follows:

Speech	*Language*
Phonetics	Grammar, Semantics

Under the heading of speech disorders, in its broadest sense, then, were placed any disturbances arising out of damage to the motor functions of the vocal organs—disorders in the anatomy, physiology or neurology of the systems concerned. In this general sense, disorders of voice production (see p. 173), fluency (see p.166) and articulation (see p. 180) could all be subsumed as 'speech disorders', as in no case was the formulation of meaning affected, but only its transmission through the medium of sound.[2] Under the heading of language disorders were grouped those disturbances which affected the formulation and comprehension of meaning—aphasia in particular (see p. 138), and also a wide range of developmental and psychological disorders.

There are several things wrong with this distinction. First, it gives exclusive emphasis to sound as a medium of communication, as opposed to the visual or tactile media—an understandable emphasis, of course (see p. 7), but a theoretically restricting one. Secondly, it apparently gives priority to the motor disorders of communication, as opposed to the sensory ones. Why is not hearing mentioned, as being a category of disability

[1] The casual use of this distinction is in fact the first 'careless practice' inveighed against by the standard text, *Diagnostic methods in speech pathology*, by W. Johnson, F. L. Darley and D. C. Spriestersbach (New York, Harper & Row 1963), 16.

[2] Sometimes a more restricted definition would be given to the notion of 'speech disorder', excluding for example the range of voice disorders: in this tradition, one would thus talk of 'voice, speech and language'. There is also a much broader definition: see below.

comparable in generality to speech, in the above sense?[3] Thirdly, there is a confusion because of the everyday meaning of the term 'speech' to mean 'spoken language'—in which, inevitably, meaning is involved. Some textbooks on disability in fact use the term in this general sense, and thus constitute a quite different tradition from that referred to above.[4] Fourthly, there is considerable uncertainty over how to apply the model in several clinical conditions. This happens especially when the disorders in question involve the phonological component of language. Phonology is 'mid-way' between phonetics and the other levels of language organization (see p. 41). It has in fact often been called a 'bridge level' or 'interlevel'. Because it constitutes the sound system of the language, it is thus intimately connected with the transmission of meaning: the fact that *pin* and *bin* are different in meaning is a consequence of the phonological opposition that distinguishes the words; and a similar point can be made about the nonsegmental aspects of phonology (though here the relationship between sound and meaning is at times even more direct, as when we talk of the emotional role of intonation in speech). On the other hand, this level is intimately connected with phonetics, i.e. with the physical realization of sound through the use of the vocal organs. There are, we have seen (p. 41) a wide range of possible realizations for a given phonological contrast, depending on the vagaries of our individual pronunciation habits. So the question is: how are we to classify disorders of the phonological system, whether segmental or nonsegmental? Are they disorders of speech or of language?

The obvious answer would seem to be, 'both', or 'don't know'. But whenever a question is unanswerable in this way, it is usually because the terms in which the question has been put are in some way irrelevant. Phonological disorders form a unique class, in linguistic pathology; they should not be identified with the meaning-generating levels of language, nor should they be identified with the phonetic manifestations of language. Disorders of intonation, for example, or dyspraxia of speech (see p. 153),

Spoken language	Phonetic disorders	Phonological disorders		
Written language	Graphetic disorders	Graphological disorders	Grammatical disorders	Semantic disorders

Fig. 32 Main categories of linguistic pathology

[3] The answer, of course, lies in the professional boundaries between speech therapist and teacher of the deaf, which have forced a division between the two sides of communication that has no theoretical justification. A teacher of the deaf has to be concerned with production, and a speech therapist with hearing. Any model of language pathology has to reflect these interdependencies, and might (it is to be hoped) suggest ways in which a measure of integration between the professions might be achieved.

[4] For example, M. F. Berry and J. Eisenson, *Speech disorders* (London, Owen 1962), which includes chapters on aphasia, language delay, etc.—and also hearing.

being primarily phonological problems, therefore do not fit easily under the original headings of speech or language—and this is perhaps why they have been the focus of controversy in recent years. A more satisfactory model of linguistic pathology will therefore be more along the lines of Fig. 4 (p. 47), as re-presented in Fig. 32: The term 'spoken language', in this respect, is far more illuminating than 'speech', and preserves a useful parallelism with other media (cf. 'written language').

Language deviance v. language delay

This is a classification of a rather different order, as it is generally applied only to cases of disorders in the acquisition of language by children. The term 'deviant' is here being used in a much narrower sense from that commonly encountered in language pathology. In its broadest sense, 'deviant' can be applied to *any* pathology, by definition—i.e., it means no more than 'abnormal'. In the present context, however, it has a more restricted application, referring to the child's use of structures, pronunciations, words etc. which are outside the normal patterns of development in children (and, one might add, which are also outside the normal range of adult possibilities for the dialect). For example, a child who said or wrote *man the* would be illustrating linguistic deviance, as this is not a possible or expected structure in the contexts just described. Similarly, a child who pronounced /h/ sounds as /k/ sounds would again be considered deviant, as this is not one of the normal substitution processes involved in language acquisition (cf. p. 180). Or again, a child who passed through the various stages of increasing complexity of language acquisition, but in the wrong order, would also be classed as deviant. Against this, there is the notion of language 'delay', where the suggestion is that everything the child says is a normal developmental feature of his language; it is simply that a time-lapse has taken place—the child should have been at that stage of development several months or years before. The delay may be in his pronunciation, his grammar, his semantics, or in some combination of these three. An alternative way of putting it is that his language is still 'immature', for his age.

   This is quite a useful distinction, but as with the others reviewed in this chapter, it must not be adopted uncritically. Let us consider the notion of deviance. This is not a homogeneous notion: there are many degrees and kinds of deviance, as we move from the area designated as 'normal'. Let us take, for example, a child's use of the /t/ phoneme in English. In a group of patients, a whole range of sounds might be substituted for the [t] which one would normally expect. A fairly predictable type of substitution is [k]—the child says /kin/ for /tin/, and so on. Rather less predictable is [p], but we can at least see some possible reasons for the confusion (they are both voiceless plosives). Less predictable still is [s], [w], and [h]—but at least these are all sounds from the same dialect. Quite inexplicable would be a sound from outside the child's dialect and apparently having nothing in common with [t]—such as the uvular trilled *r* (as in French). There are evidently degrees of deviance between these substitutions, though it is not always possible to give reasons as to why one sound should be more or less deviant than another. And a similar argument applies to a child's deviant use of grammar or vocabulary. Which of the following two deviant sentences would you say was the more deviant?

cat the on be mat
going to the boy play

It is extremely difficult to decide; and deviant sentences, therefore, often have to remain unanalysed in a grammatical analysis of language disorders.

There are also complications within the notion of delay. If you take this notion literally, then the category probably does not exist. A 'delayed' child of seven years of age would be interpreted to mean that he is displaying *exactly* the range of linguistic habits you would expect to see in a younger child. This would mean that not only the qualitative range of his language reflected this less mature norm, but also the quantity of language would be that characteristic of the younger group. This rarely, if ever, happens. What we find is several different kinds of 'unbalanced' language delay—a delay which is mainly located under the heading of pronunciation, or of grammar, or of vocabulary—and if, say, grammar, then affecting certain aspects of grammar more than others (see further, p. 163). If the child was psychologically normal, he would also be wanting to 'do' several things with his language which the younger child would not be doing, and this would add further differences. In diagnosing such children, therefore, an important step is the drawing up of as complete a profile of their linguistic abilities as possible, to establish to what extent and in what areas of language there are genuine delays. And in the course of doing this, we may well encounter deviance as well as delay—a 'mixed' category of patient, once again.

Abnormal v. normal

Underlying much of this discussion is an assumption which itself is not immune from criticism—the idea that it is possible to draw a clear dividing-line between the concepts of normality and abnormality. Of course, this is a distinction with which everyone attempts to work, despite the unhappy overtones which the term 'abnormal' often connotes. (Nor is there any necessary implication of pathology: abnormality may mean simply idiosyncrasy, eccentricity, or brilliance.) There is likely to be a gradient between the two (as already seen, in the notion of deviance), and the decision as to whether a behaviour is normal or abnormal will often be very difficult to make, especially where psychological problems are involved. The analyst's views may be different from those of the patient, and different analysts may have different views. The point is a real one, as (in a more sophisticated form) it arises every time a decision has to be made as to whether a child should attend a special school (cf. p. 130) or an adult be consigned to an institution. But there are certain useful guidelines to be obtained from a consideration of this distinction.

Firstly, the concept of the abnormal is plainly dependent on some kind of prior recognition being given to the notion of normal. (cf. p. 10) One would not teach ENT pathology on a speech therapy course, for instance, until a basic understanding of the normal anatomy and physiology had been established. But this point is not quite as obvious as it sounds, when it comes to linguistic studies. Let us imagine an 'abnormal' child turning up at a clinic. An assessment must be carried out, and the nature of the abnormality pinpointed. But with what norm should he be compared? How *should* he be speaking? The therapist will need to know the dialect the child comes from, in case there are differences between the way she speaks and the way the child will be expected to speak by his parents and peers. She will need to know how much language he should have acquired for his age—and also for his sex (in some areas of language, the rate of acquisition of girls is faster than that of boys) and social background (there are differences in the expectations parents have about their children's language, and this may relate to differences in social class).[5] She will need to know how rapidly children of his age (sex, etc.) generally pick up new language—so that she can evaluate whether his response to language treatment is normal. She will need to know the norms of mother-child interaction, so that in her choice of language to use to the child, she does not introduce structures, words, and so on that are going to be wholly unfamiliar to him. And (as there is no knowing in advance how old a patient is going to be, before he turns up) she must anticipate being able to provide this normative information for all ages of development, up to and including the adult language. It is the adult language which provides the terminus for her work, and this must be thoroughly understood, if she is to be able to decide on a remedial programme which will ultimately reach that goal. Only one principle seems valid, in clinical analysis: that anything that *can* go wrong, linguistically, *will*, sooner or later, in some patient! One must therefore be in total command of the field of language studies, and always expect the unexpected.

If only we were all in the position of having fully mastered these norms! Unfortunately, the real world is a long way away from the ideals of the previous paragraph. Some norms are fairly well established (e.g. grammatical norms of development up to age four, or so), but others have received little scientific study (e.g. the detailed differences between rates of development for boys and girls). And the more 'exceptional' the patient, the less likely there will be information about norms. As soon as we consider the special problems of immigrants, bilinguals, physically handicapped, and other 'abnormal' groups, the size of the problem should be apparent. Even in the field of local dialect, there are great gaps in our information. How

[5] See J. R. Edwards, *Language and disadvantage* (London, Edward Arnold 1979).

children acquire the sounds and grammatical structures of southern British English is well written up; but there are few formal clinical studies on children from Scotland, Yorkshire, Birmingham, Northern Ireland . . . It is here that clinical applications of such fields as sociolinguistics (cf. p. 47) would be most welcome.

As each attempt at a general classification of linguistic disorders is reviewed, the same story repeats itself. Several very astute insights into the nature of disability have become formalized as clinical categories, on the basis of very little evidence. The main difficulty in the way of progress is the paucity of empirical studies, and (until recently) the lack of a method of investigation capable of identifying the disorders in behavioural terms. In my view, we are now in a position where the second of these problems is solved: several linguistic methods are available to get the work done. Unfortunately, the time and opportunity for clinically-qualified people to carry out the required empirical work is not easy to find. Progress therefore remains slow, and the traditional categories and terminology continue to be used, in the absence of anything more constructive to emerge from the newer approaches. Perhaps the best we can do, under the circumstances, is investigate the range of linguistic pathologies, within the traditional frame of reference, but with an open and critical mind. At all points, we must remember that to label a disability is not to provide an explanation. If a child has problems with pronouncing [s], we have added little to our understanding of his difficulty by labelling his problem a 'sigmatism'. Rather, a label should be supported by a set of *criteria of analysis*, which will systematically differentiate the disorder from others with which it is likely to be confused, and explain the internal variability which can be found within the disorder. This is why I pay so much attention to descriptive terminology, throughout the following pages, and why I keep stressing the limitations of our present state of knowledge. I hope that, by my doing this, at least some of the readers of this book will feel motivated to aim to do some research in the field, and thus contribute to the broadening of its knowledge base, which it so badly needs.

In the rest of this chapter, I shall review the main characteristics of the major categories of linguistic pathology. I shall follow the general direction of the communication chain, but shall begin, this time, with disorders of input (deafness), leading on to 'central' disorders involving language (aphasia, and other conditions), and then to the range of output disorders (fluency, voice, articulation). I shall conclude with a few general remarks about the field as a whole.

Pathologies of reception

Deafness
In 1977, the Royal National Institute for the Deaf began yet another publicity campaign to bring home to the public at large the devastating

effects of deafness on human beings, and the need for greater levels of public sympathy and understanding. Slogans such as 'Mind that child; he may be deaf' illustrate the essence of the problem, and the uniqueness of this pathology: deafness is a condition which cannot be seen. The need for a special understanding of this problem is thus apparent. The extent of the pathology is often underestimated: in a recent report, it was estimated that in 1975 there were 170,000 children (under 16) and 2,360,000 adults suffering from some degree of hearing loss in Great Britain.[6]

This formulation immediately raises a theoretical problem: the distinction between *deafness* and *hearing loss*. Given the nature of the auditory apparatus and its acoustic input (see Chapter 3), it will be plain that loss of hearing is not a single homogeneous category. The contrast between being deaf (unable to respond to sound) and being 'not deaf' is never clearcut. Rather there is a potentially infinite range of degrees of hearing loss, ranging from a very slight inability to respond to a few low-intensity frequencies (which will hardly interfere with normal communication) to a loss where there is no detectable response to any frequency no matter how intense the sound. This latter condition we would obviously want to call 'deaf', but it is in fact fairly uncommon: the vast majority of people diagnosed as deaf do have some degree of response to sound (they have some 'residual hearing'). Most people, in other words, are spread over the scale of hearing loss, in a way which makes it impossible to draw anything other than the grossest of distinctions. But distinctions have to be drawn.[7] For young children suffering from hearing loss, decisions must be made as to how they are to be educated. In Britain, various types of institution are available: there are special *schools for the deaf*, which cater for the more severely handicapped child; there are a few *schools for the partially-hearing*; and there are *partially hearing units*, usually attached to normal schools, which cater for the less handicapped. Partially-hearing children are also often placed in normal classes, receiving special assistance from a peripatetic teacher of the deaf. Unfortunately, it is not always obvious which type of institution will best meet the needs of the child with a considerable, but not particularly severe degree of hearing loss; a lot depends on the use the child is making of whatever hearing is available to him; and it is in such circumstances that the theoretical problems of defining deafness become practical and social ones.

Investigating hearing loss involves three interrelated decisions: where is the cause of the deafness located? how great is the degree of hearing loss? and what type of hearing loss is it? The otologist is responsible for the first of these questions (cf. above, p. 119); the person responsible for the other two is the *audiologist. Audiology* is the study of hearing and its disorders. It is specifically concerned with assessing the nature and degree of hearing loss

---

[6] Department of Health and Social Security report (June 1977) by the Advisory Committee on Services for Hearing-Impaired People.

[7] For example, one system of classification distinguishes degrees of hearing impairment as follows: mild—loss of 27–40 dB; moderate—loss of 41–55 dB; moderately severe—loss of 56–70 dB; severe—loss of 71–90 dB; profound—loss of 91 + dB.

and conservation, and with the rehabilitation of people with hearing impairment. When the focus is on children, the specialized techniques involved are known as *pediatric audiology*. *Audiometry* is the scientific measurement of hearing, using, in particular, the audiometer (cf. p. 113). A wide range of *audiometric tests* is available, to determine the nature and degree of hearing sensitivity. One of the most widely used techniques is *pure-tone audiometry*, which uses a specially calibrated machine to generate pure tones at different frequencies and intensities; these are presented to the patient one ear at a time through headphones (in an *air-conduction* test), or through the bone behind each ear (in a *bone-conduction* test). The patient indicates when he senses a sound, and the results are plotted as an audiogram; (see Fig. 33; cf. Fig. 29). *Speech audiometry* aims to obtain a measure of the patient's response to speech, as opposed to pure-tone stimuli. It may be carried out impressionistically, with the audiologist speaking at different levels and distances from the patient; but a more precise estimate can be achieved by recording a series of words or sentences representing the various kinds of speech sound and playing these back to the patient at known intensities under various conditions.

Using these techniques, in the context of the anatomical, physiological and neurological conditions outlined above, one can make a major differential diagnosis of hearing loss into two broad categories, based primarily on where the lesions occur in the auditory pathway: *conductive* deafness and *sensorineural* (or *neural*, or *nerve*) deafness. Conductive deafness refers to any interference with the transmission of sound to the inner ear; sensorineural deafness refers to interference arising from the inner ear itself, or in that part of the auditory nerve as far back as its first synapse in the brain stem. Sensorineural deafness is further divided into the common *sensory* (or *cochlear*) deafness, due to inner ear damage, and the rarer *neural* deafness, due to VIII nerve disease, typically a tumour (*acoustic neuroma*). Figure 33(a) illustrates a case of moderate conductive deafness; there is a fairly uniform reduction in intensity throughout the frequency range. This might have been caused by any of the outer/middle ear problems outlined in Chapter 3. A case of sensorineural deafness is illustrated in Figure 33(b): here, the patient has had particular difficulty responding to the high frequencies ('high tone deafness'), indicating that there has been some specific damage to the receptor cells in the organ of Corti which handle those frequencies, or to those nerve fibres which transmit these frequencies to the brain. An important factor in the diagnosis will be the ability of the patient to respond differentially to air-conduction and bone-conduction tests (the audiograms in Fig. 33 were air-conduction only). If he cannot hear sounds through the air, but can hear them through his skull, it suggests that a conductive deafness is present; conversely, if there is no difference in his hearing between these two modes, the damage must be neural. More complex, 'mixed' cases of deafness also occur.

A specific example of (fluctuating) neural deafness occurs in *Ménière's*

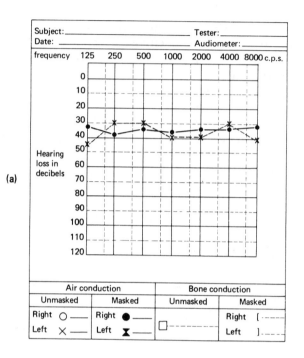

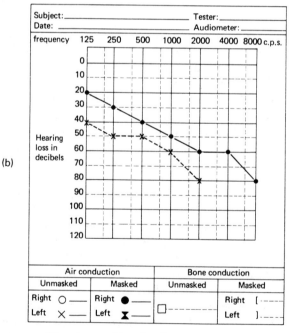

Fig. 33 Audiograms of two types of hearing loss:
(a) conductive deafness; (b) sensorineural deafness

disease (discovered by the French physician, Prosper Ménière, in 1861), along with tinnitus, giddiness (*vertigo*, a disorder of the vestibular nerve) and vomiting. *Tinnitus* itself is little understood: it refers to noises in the ear, which may take on several different qualities—ringing, buzzing, hissing, pulsating. . . . Most of us have experienced a mild tinnitus (e.g. 'ringing in the ears'), and any slightly abnormal condition, such as excessive wax, might produce it. But it often occurs in acute form (as in Ménière's disease), in which the noise levels can be desperately irritating and painful—a condition which the sufferer can only learn to live with, by attempting to ignore it or mask it in some way. It is generally felt that the cause lies deep within the cochlea, but the reason for the specific qualities of sound (e.g. whether the cochlea is in some way picking up sounds from the circulation of the blood) is unknown.

Conductive and sensorineural deafness are sometimes grouped together under the more general heading of *peripheral deafness*, and opposed to the little-understood phenomenon of *central* (or *cortical*) *deafness*. Central deafness refers to the loss of hearing sensitivity due to damage of the auditory nerve in the brain stem or in the hearing centres of the cortex (cf. p. 84). It is sometimes referred to as 'auditory imperception', and this term illustrates the issue that is involved: the ear seems normal, as can be shown by a pure-tone audiogram, which will produce normal results; but the patient will respond poorly to speech audiometry, being unable to integrate and interpret the sounds of speech. The problem of diagnosis here, of course, is in deciding whether this is purely an auditory problem, or whether a more fundamental linguistic pathology is involved (as in Wernicke's aphasia, see p. 151), or something even more deep-rooted (as with the failure to respond of severely autistic children, see p. 159).

Other variables may enter into the classification of hearing loss. Apart from the above distinctions, we must obviously allow for 'mixed' types of deafness, in which both conductive and neural elements are involved. This is particularly noticeable as part of the natural process of hearing loss associated with age (*presbycusis*): sounds become fainter, generally, but with certain sounds (usually the consonants involving the higher frequencies) causing particular problems. Speech will get through, but it will be full of 'gaps'; it will thus take much longer to interpret, and it is this which accounts for the slow response of many old people to speech, even when it is shouted (shouting will usually not help: what they need is *time* to decode the partially-received signal). Unfortunately, such slow responses are often interpreted as a diminution in the person's mental faculties—which is by no means necessarily the case.

An important further distinction is whether one or both ears is involved. If the problem affects only one ear, it is referred to as *monaural* or *unilateral*; if two ears, it is *binaural* or *bilateral*. It is usual to refer to a patient's hearing abilities with reference to his 'better ear', if he has one.

Yet another distinction to note is that between *congenital* and *acquired* deafness. The former means 'present at birth', insofar as this can be established, and usually subsumes cases of genetic origin as well as those where the deafness was caused by disease or trauma in the womb or during birth itself. Acquired, or *adventitious* deafness, refers to the later onset of this disorder, as a result of disease or trauma, throughout the whole period of child and adult life. In relation to this distinction, three points should be stressed: (a) The need for routine auditory screening at or shortly after birth is paramount, but is infrequently carried out. Over 95 per cent of the babies born deaf have some degree of residual hearing, and the earlier that auditory training can be established with such children, the better the prognosis for the later development of speech. (b) An important issue, in relation to acquired deafness, is whether the change took place before or after the onset for the learning of language. If some language input has taken place before the advent of the deafness, the teacher of the deaf is much helped in the attempt to facilitate the language learning process. (c) If deafness is congenital, or acquired in the first months of life, when will it be first noticed? One factor to remember here is that deaf infants do cry, coo and babble in the early months of life; they do not remain silent. Studies are few, but those that have been made suggest that there is considerable variation in the early babble of deaf infants, though it tends to be less in quantity and (as time passes) less purposeful than with hearing infants. By the end of the first year of life, some indication of the presence of deafness is normally present in the 'flattened' tones of the child's babble, compared with the developing intonation of hearing children, which will become more and more language-specific as time goes by. It is possible to begin telling the language backgrounds of infants apart, on the basis of their early babbling and attempts at speech, from as early as 9 months; and it is from this time, accordingly, that a phonetic analysis (of nonsegmental vocal effect, cf. p. 41) might be able to contribute to diagnosis.

Later work with the deaf is a complex and time-consuming business. There are of course a variety of aids available, but it should be noted that as a rule hearing-aids only amplify sound presented to the ear—they cannot help in the interpretation of that sound. Moreover, *all* sound in the environment of the person may be amplified—including the background noises to speech. Lip-reading skills also constitute an important additional aid to comprehension. But what about speech production? The difficulty which deaf children have in learning to speak is well illustrated by the traditional (and misleading) term, 'deaf and dumb'. The term is misleading because it does not at all follow that if you are deaf you will be unable to speak. Everything depends on the kind of deafness involved, the amount and quality of your exposure to speech, the kind of teaching you receive, and so on. But it is a fact that, for whatever reason, most congenitally deaf people grow up with a functionally inadequate speech level, i.e. they cannot produce intelligible speech for the whole range of occasions where they want to communicate. Partly as a result of the apparent failure of this mode of language learning, many teachers of the deaf in recent years have focused their attention on the possibility of teaching the deaf to communicate by means of developing their natural *signing* capacities. All of us have an ability to gesture our meaning, on occasion, but the range of meanings which we can signal in this way is very limited. In so-called *sign languages*, however, a range of several thousand meanings can be communicated, and whole communities of the deaf have learned to use these systems. Some of these systems have developed naturally, from within the deaf communities (such as American Sign Language (ASL), or British Sign Language). Others have been artificially constructed to meet a particular purpose (such as the Paget-Gorman Sign System, which attempts to reflect in its sign sequences the grammatical rules of English sentences).[8]

Other forms of signing behaviour have been devised to help the deaf. *Finger-spelling* (or *dactyology*) provides a manual alphabet (there are both one-handed and two-handed versions) which enables anyone to spell out words on their fingers. The alphabet used by the British Deaf Association is illustrated in Fig. 34. Then there is *cued speech*, a system devised by Orin Cornett, an American researcher in deaf education at Gallaudet University, Washington; this supplements the movements of the lips by a series of signals representing some of the main sound contrasts involved in speech, thereby aiding the deaf person's comprehension. And there are many other schemes. Reaction to all forms of *manual* communication has been mixed, over the years. Indeed, in the world of the deaf, it is commonplace to find educators who are fiercely in favour of signing (so-called 'manualists') and those who are fiercely against it (so-called 'oralists'). There are also others who try to make use of both systems of communication in their work. The arguments on both sides are important and far-reaching, but are often obscured because of the emotion which is engendered when the issue is discussed. The main argument against signing is that it is setting the deaf person apart from all but his own small community, labelling him as deaf and different, and not helping him in his desire to communicate with the outside world. To which argument the manualist might well respond that this is no worse than the situation which exists for the deaf person who has been trained in an oralist tradition: he cannot communicate with the outside world either, and is readily labelled as deaf, on account of his absent or unintelligible speech. A manual system of communication is a positive gain, he might argue, for people who have nothing else, and it is moreover capable of providing a very wide range of communicative experience in social and artistic life. To which the oralist might respond that the weaknesses in oral methods can be circumvented by the development of new techniques of language teaching, such as the devices now available for displaying features of the voice visually (e.g. the *laryngograph*, which makes the larynx

---

[8] The system was invented by Sir Richard Paget, and developed by his wife after his death, in collaboration with the librarian of the RNID in London, Pierre Gorman. It was published in 1976 as *The Paget Gorman Sign System Manual* (London, Association for Experiment in Deaf Education Ltd.).

frequency visible, and thus motivates the deaf person to improve his voice pitch). And so the argument continues. When such matters as a person's identity and the fullness of his life enter into an argument, it is evident why emotions are easily roused. But one fact cannot be obscured by the arguments of both sides—the pressing need for research into all aspects of deaf communicative behaviour. What stages of language do deaf children pass through as they begin their acquisition process? To what extent do deaf

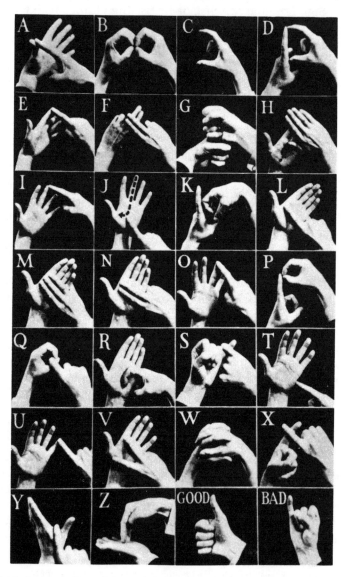

Fig. 34 British finger-spelling alphabet (© The British Deaf Association)

children develop a system of their own, when learning language—a kind of 'deafish', as it has sometimes been called? Which structures of the adult language cause particular problems of comprehension for the deaf, whether child or adult? Are there limits to the amount of visual discrimination, which might affect the learning of a sign system? These and many other questions remain to be investigated systematically.[9]

To illustrate the kind of linguistic problems encountered in analysing the language of deaf children, four samples of their free writing (the first two in response to a picture stimulus) are given below. The first (A) is from a 12½-year-old girl, whose audiogram is given in Figure 35(a).

The guinea pig

There is a guinea pig. The guinea pig name is Funny. The guinea pig got black and white. The guinea pig got pink nose. The guinea pig is standing. The guinea pig is waiting the food. The guinea pig got pink ears. The guinea pig got four leg. The guinea pig is standing on the table. The guinea pig look at the boy.

The second is from a 14½-year-old boy (B), whose audiogram is given in Figure 35(b).

White horse

There is a white horse in a forest he has large ears and big brown eyes. He have got lots of hair all over his eye on one side. His nostrils are about 2 cm wide. He is very wild horse. The forest are black the grass are nice and green. He has got a brown harness. Sometime he ran away and eat people apple in the garden. His eyes looks as they are coming out.

Several of the deaf child's linguistic difficulties are illustrated by these extracts. There is an extremely restricted range of sentence structure, most noticeable in the stereotyped sentence openings in the guinea-pig story. There are problems with articles (*He is very wild horse*), tenses (*Sometime he ran . . . and eat*), prepositions (*is waiting the food*), agreement between subject and verb (*he have . . ., the forest are . . .*), omission of auxiliary verbs (*the guinea pig look at*), and omission of certain word-endings (*the guinea pig name*). It is sometimes difficult to be sure what sentence is intended: how, for example, would you correct A's third sentence—*The guinea pig is black and white*? or *. . . has a black and white coat*? The third extract illustrates this problem in extreme form. It was written by a 16½-year-old boy whose audiogram is given in Figure 35(c). The analysis of this kind of language presents major problems to the language pathologist, whose aim is to establish how much of this data has an underlying pattern. It also illustrates the need for as early intervention as possible with such children, with the aim of teaching a stable basis of linguistic structure, and thus preventing the development of such ungrammatical sequences.

[9] For further discussion of deafness, see J. Ballantyne, *Deafness* (London, Churchill Livingstone, 3rd edn, 1977), E. Whetnall and D. B. Fry, *The deaf child* (London, Heinemann 1971), H. Davis and S. R. Silverman (eds), *Hearing and deafness* (New York, Holt, Rinehart & Winston, 3rd edn., 1970).

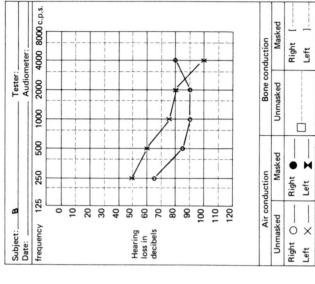

Subject: A   Tester:
Date: Audiometer:

frequency 125 250 500 1000 2000 4000 8000 c.p.s.

Hearing loss in decibels: 0 to 120

Air conduction		Bone conduction	
Unmasked	Masked	Unmasked	Masked
Right ○	Right ●		Right [
Left ✕	Left ✖	☐	Left]

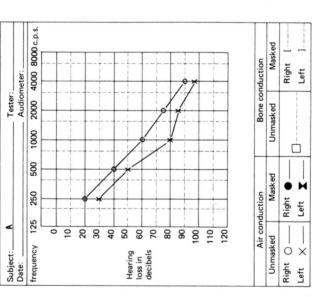

Subject: B   Tester:
Date: Audiometer:

frequency 125 250 500 1000 2000 4000 8000 c.p.s.

Hearing loss in decibels: 0 to 120

Air conduction		Bone conduction	
Unmasked	Masked	Unmasked	Masked
Right ○	Right ●		Right [
Left ✕	Left ✖	☐	Left]

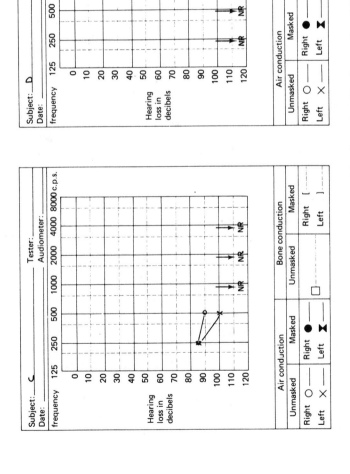

Fig. 35 Audiograms of the four children whose writing is analysed in the text (pp. 137, 140)

Star Wars
The Star Wars was the two spaceship a fighting opened door was coming the Men and Storm trooper guns carry on to Artoo Detoo and threepio at go the space. The Earth was not grass and tree but to the sand, R2D2 and C3P0 at going look for R2D2 walk the sand people carry away Artoo Detoo sleep. The Luke Skywalker Came was van Horrible and the his was Came C3P0 to walked the to R2D2 the Man said No and to other one Small Came was bomb as no good. The C3P0 ask to man was oh! yes with came to R2D2 yes very good. The R2D2 going long away the his said C3P0 as the Nobody was long away as the his bring Binoculars For Look round not they was the car float as but the very fast and you are found R2D2. The spaceship to away the Earth space-metal the long away very big Earth.

A much more satisfactory outcome is illustrated by the fourth extract, from a 16¼-year-old girl (D), whose audiogram is given in Figure 35(d).

Snow
It was Saturday morning. I woke up and I got dress. Then I drew the curtain.
I looked through the window and found that everything was white and the water had changed into ice. I sat down on a chair by the window.
I was looking everywhere. On the long lake beside my house was a small white bridge and under the bridge were a long icicle drop. The drop had made a small hole in the frozen lake. In the small hole, I could see two little fishes swimming about. The lake looked like glass with a small hole in it.
The grass was cover in snow and it looked like a very big white carpet with some footmark. I didn't know who made the footmark. I was thinking who come to my door and goes back again. I follow the footmark to see if I get any clue. Then I found there were three bottles of milk so I thought it must be the milkman.

'Central' pathologies

When investigating disorders of language which originate in the central nervous system, it is usual to distinguish two broad categories: (a) those where the linguistic problems appear to be the result of organic pathology in specific centres of the brain (especially those listed on p. 84 above), in which language is the primary or the only aspect of behaviour affected; and (b) those where the linguistic problem is plainly a reflex of an underlying psychological disturbance of unclear etiology. The first category is known as *aphasia*. The second has no specific name for the linguistic disturbance, the symptoms concerned being considered along with other, nonlinguistic symptoms within the field of psychopathology. In between, there is a grey area of mixed disorders, displaying both linguistic and psychological elements, and varying degrees of organic pathology, which are sometimes grouped under the heading of aphasia, in a broad interpretation for this term, and sometimes taken separately.

Aphasia
We may begin with this uncertainty of definition, as it reflects a basic controversy within the field of *aphasiology*. The broad definition of aphasia permits any difficulty a patient has with 'symbolic' function as a result of

brain damage to be placed under this heading. According to the British neurologist, Henry Head, for example, aphasia was a disorder of 'symbolic formulation and expression'.[10] Language, being the main means of symbolic expression, would be centrally affected; but so would other forms of behaviour involving symbols, e.g. the ability to see analogies between objects, understand traffic signs, make colour associations, interpret gestures. There would also be changes in the intellectual capacities of the *aphasic* (or *dysphasic*) patient,[11] such as his ability to remember, draw logical conclusions, perform arithmetical operations, or pay attention. There would be a general reduction in his efficiency, e.g. he would tire more easily. He may have problems in coordinating different aspects of his behaviour, e.g. relating what he sees to movements of his hand ('hand-eye' coordination). He may also undergo personality changes, perhaps becoming more irritable, emotional or depressive. Given these characteristics, seen in many patients, it was difficult to see aphasia as constituting purely a linguistic disorder. At the very least, it seemed to involve a more deeprooted incapacity to use symbols (*asymbolia*), and cognitive and personality problems as well.

A more specific conception of aphasia defines it solely as a linguistic pathology: a recent dictionary of communicative disorders, for example, sees it as a 'communication disorder caused by brain damage and character-ized by complete or partial impairment of language comprehension, formu-lation, and use'.[12] The definition continues: aphasia 'excludes disorders associated with primary sensory deficits, general mental deterioration, or psychiatric disorders'—and, we might add, primary motor deficits as well (see further, p. 155). On this account, therefore, we are exclusively within the area of language, and we will allow for the possibility that the dysphasic patient will be very much the same as he was before, in all respects bar his reduced ability in speaking, comprehending, reading or writing. His disturbances here would then be analysable into the recognized categories of language—syntax, semantics, phonology and so on.

In the final analysis, the difference between the two approaches, and the many other overlapping definitions of aphasia which exist, may reduce to one of emphasis. Perhaps both are right; perhaps their authors are thinking of different kinds of dysphasic patient, or patients at different stages of treatment or recovery? Certainly, this is the main impression that hits anyone entering this field of study for the first time—the bewildering variety of pathological behaviours that are presented by people who have suffered

[10] H. Head, *Aphasia and kindred disorders of speech* (Cambridge, CUP 1926).

[11] In theory, the change of prefix carries with it a difference of meaning: *a-* means 'total lack of'; *dys-* means 'partial lack of'. In practice, because there are few cases where a total absence of language is the result of the pathology, a general usage has grown up in which a patient suffering from aphasia is called 'dysphasic'. In the United States, the term 'aphasic' is nonetheless the normal form. What is important is to realize that there is normally no change of meaning between the two terms. If the *complete* loss of language needs to be stressed, then a phrase such as 'completely aphasic' will be used.

[12] L. Nicolosi, E. Harryman and J. Kresheck, *Terminology of communication disorders* (Baltimore, Williams & Wilkins 1978), 9.

from brain damage. No two patients seem identical, as far as their linguistic and cognitive faculties are concerned. And this turns out to be more than just a first impression, as detailed analysis of patient samples shows the differences to be considerable. This should not be surprising; when we recall the vast extent of brain cells which may be damaged (cf. p. 79), large individual differences are only to be expected. As a result, it is at least possible that many of the differences between the several theoretical positions taken up concerning aphasia are the result of sampling and methodological differences on the part of the analysts. It is wise, accordingly, to adopt a fairly flexible position at the outset—expecting linguistic problems to be the primary symptoms, but not excluding the possibility of important deficiencies in memory, attention, logical sequencing, and other such areas.

Notwithstanding the many individual differences, it is usual to try to classify aphasic behaviour into broad types. Most of these attempts have ended up with a binary classification, some of the pairs of terms being as follows:

expressive	receptive
executive	evaluative
production	comprehension
motor	sensory
encoding	decoding
Broca's	Wernicke's
nonfluent	fluent

The main aim behind these terms is to produce a classification which makes sense from both neurological and behavioural points of view. The motor/sensory contrast is well-established neurologically, as is the distinction between Broca's and Wernicke's areas (cf. p. 84); the production/comprehension contrast is well-established psychologically, as is the contrast between encoding and decoding. The expressive/receptive terminology subsumes aspects of both these emphases, and it is perhaps for this reason that these terms have achieved widespread use. Dysphasics are, accordingly, said to have difficulties in the expression (formulation, production, encoding) of language, or with its reception (decoding, comprehension). These days, it is emphasized in textbooks that such terms are not absolutes, representing a clearcut division. Rather, when we refer to a dysphasic as 'expressive' or 'receptive', we are doing this on the basis of his most dominant symptoms. It is rare that we encounter a patient who is 'just' expressive, i.e. his receptive abilities are wholly intact, his sole problems being with the expression of speech; and similarly, a 'just' receptive patient is also a rarity. The general rule is to talk about patients as *predominantly expressive* and *predominantly receptive*. There is also an important category where the problems seem to affect both modes more or less equally—a *mixed* (sometimes referred to as a *global*, or *central*) disorder. Some clinicians in fact feel that it is this latter state which is the most usual one—arguing for a 'unitary' or 'holistic' interpretation of aphasia, in which speech and comprehension are always affected, in varying degrees.

How can we characterize an expressive aphasic patient? Here is one sample, taken from a patient aged 47, who two years previously had suffered a CVA, arising from a complete occlusion of the left internal carotid artery; there was a right hemiplegia and a right homonymous hemianopia (cf. above, p. 85). From an originally total aphasia, he had progressed to use such language as the following:[13]

T	(*showing a picture of a cowboy lassoing a horse*) 'what's thìs/ —
P	erm —
T	mhṁ/ —
P	'cowboys * 'and —
T	*mhṁ/ — —
P	'cowboy 'and . wréstler/ — 'wrestler 'and —
T	wèll/ . the 'horse is 'tied with a rópe/ . ìsn't it/
P	a ròpe/ . 'ah 'yes yès/
T	'what are they 'doing with the ròpe/ —
	'what are they 'doing with the ròpe/
P	strīng/ .
T	ṁhm/ .
P	yēs/ — — strīng/ . strìng/
T	mhṁ/ . 'they're pùlling it/
P	pūl'ling 'it/ . 'ah yēs/ 'pu (*whispers*)
T	pùlling it/ . pùlling it/
P	yès yes/

. . .   . . .

T	'what are they dòing/ — —
P	bōy/
T	*mhṁ/ .
P	*gīrl/ .
T	mhṁ/ — 'try 'joining it ùp/ —
P	*4 syllables*
T	'ah hăh/
P	'the 'boy īs/
T	gòod/ . ṁhm/
P	'the 'boy īs — — 'the 'boy īs — . — yěs/ — yěs/
T	rìght/ yěs/ . you've gòt it/ sìtting/
P	sīngit/

The extract illustrates several typical features of expressive aphasia. Under the heading of grammar, we would note the reduced and incomplete sentence structure (what is sometimes loosely referred to as *agrammatic*

[13] Transcription conventions: increasing pause length marked by . (short), —, — — (long); each unit of intonation (cf. p. 41) is marked by /; the main pitch movement in this unit is indicated by an accent (ˋ falling, ˊ rising, ˉ level); stress on other syllables is marked by '. * indicates that the therapist was speaking at the same time as the patient. T = therapist; P = patient.

speech). Under semantics, there is the difficulty the patient has in *word-finding*, and the great reliance he places on the therapist's stimuli. He finds nouns in particular difficult to retrieve—a disability referred to as *anomia* (or *nominal* aphasia). Under the heading of phonology, we should note the uncertain and often inappropriate use of intonation (*yes yes* is often said very confidently, when in fact the patient is quite confused) and the erratic pausing. The term *dysprosody* may be used to refer to such characteristics (see also p. 174). The sample also shows some *echolalia*—repetition with minimal change of what has just been said to him, in a context which suggests that comprehension is absent. There is only one example of the inaccurate use of segmental phonemes, which can also characterize expressive aphasia: /singit/ for *sitting*. This tendency to transpose, substitute and add irrelevant sounds (though nonetheless correctly articulated) is traditionally known as *literal paraphasia*, though it would perhaps be more accurate to refer to the problem as *phonological paraphasia*.[14]

This sample also illustrates the difficulty of making a clear decision about the expressive/receptive issue. Theoretically, an expressive aphasic has good comprehension—but is this true in this instance? Or rather, how could you be sure? How would you analyse the patient's difficulties with *pulling it*, for instance? (a) Did he fully understand the phrase, but had difficulty producing it? or (b) Did he *not* fully understand the phrase, but still had difficulty in producing it? This is in fact a classical analytic problem, which can be resolved only by careful checking of the patient's comprehension skills, using a structured situation where the alternatives that the patient can respond to are completely under your control. Only then would it be possible to be sure that there was, or was not, a comprehension problem in this case. And the practical problems in the way of organizing such experimental situations are so great that often the matter is left undecided.

To illustrate the variation within the 'expressive' category, here is an extract from another patient diagnosed as predominantly expressive. This 64-year-old gentleman was admitted to a neurology ward with a transient right-sided hemiplegia and aphasia, but brain-scan showed no major abnormalities. The following recording was made a month later.

T   how've you been getting òn/
P   yés/ been going alríght/ yés/ lóvely/ yés/ thánk you/
T   had a game of gólf since I last saw you/
P   nó/ (*2 syllables*) Sŭnday/ on ?a Súnday/ that's ăll/ nó/ . nó/ ànyway/ next Sùnday/ ànyway/
T   nèxt Sunday/
P   yéah/ I (*2 syllábles*)/ yés/

[14] The term 'paraphasia' is a general term, which refers in its broadest sense to any error involving the unintentional substitution, transposition or addition of a basic unit of language—whether sound, syllable, morpheme or word, in either speech or writing. The important point is that this label suggests that the patient's phonological system is fundamentally disordered—lacking certain phonemes, or the rules governing their organization. The contrast is with dyspraxia (cf. p. 153), where the phonological system is felt to be intact, but not under the control of the patient.

T   why can't you play during the wèek/
P   wèll/ it's—it's Jŏhn/ . it's for the càr/ sèe/ . it's for the car it's — it's got too far awày sée/
T   oh I sèe/ so your son . drìves you/
P   thàt's right/ yéah/
T   *mhm̀/
P   *and the . cár/ . and the and the and the . whatsisname and the and . they give the . whàtisname you sée/ . so . other thăn/ . there's no gòod . sée/ .
T   *yèah/
P   *well it's nò good/ . will a bús/ get me . clúbs/ and all thát/*(   )* dòn't it/ rĕally/
T   *oh you can't get on a bùs/*
    do you not know any ôther people who play golf/ who could play in the wèek/
P   nò/ I'm afraid . I'm afràid not/ rèally not —/not nobody over there with er — with the pèople/ rèally/ ŏtherwise/ I I'd lìke to/ rĕally/ — ?to gò there/ rĕally/ cos it's it's/sēe/ alright/ sèe/
T   rathèr/
P   you knōw/ but er . I mèan/ er . Jóhn/ and . Éddy/ . he's at Néwbury/ he likes down thére/ and er . that's ìt/ sée/ — so they just got . real . what's thàt/ . the only thing is/ (*3 syllables*) whatisname (*2 syllables*) whatisname (*1 syllable*) whàtisname/ — (*2 syllables*) ŏtherwise/ it's only for one — Sŭnday/ and they only . it it I mean there really is sée/

This sample displays several interesting features, many of which again blur the distinction between expressive and receptive categories. Under the heading of grammar, we should note the rapidly-produced, incompletely-structured and erratically-sequenced sentences. There are several involuntary repetitions of words and phrases—a feature referred to as *palilalia* in classical speech pathology terms. Under the heading of semantics, we note several examples of unintelligible speech (or *jargon*), of talking around a subject (*circumlocution*), marked word-finding difficulties, and the fragmentation of sentence meaning into several smaller and poorly related chunks (perhaps because of a highly restricted auditory memory). A great deal of the language used is either irrelevant, empty of meaning, or lacking in comprehension, and it is this underlying tendency which makes it difficult to extract the intended meaning from his utterances. The therapist is doing very well, under the circumstances, in keeping the conversation going![15] Under the heading of phonology, we would note, for this patient, a generally confident, boisterous tone, punctuated by frequent hesitations—an inappropriate tone, of course, given his difficulties. A general tendency, which can affect grammar, vocabulary or phonology, is *perseveration*—a tendency for the patient to continue an activity once begun, so that he is unable to stop it, even though it is no longer appropriate to continue. This kind of automatic, involuntary continuation of behaviour can be seen on *really* and *whatsisname* in the above sample.

[15] If we ignore the irrelevance and emptiness in the discourse, the beginnings of coherence emerge, e.g. l. 9–10 *John—car—too far away*. The therapist's task is twofold: to establish which aspects of the speech are central to the patient's meaning, and to interrelate them into a coherent whole.

Let us turn now to an example of the other category of patient. How would we characterize a patient with a predominantly receptive aphasia? The following sample is taken from a 66-year-old male patient, six months after a left CVA, with an associated right hemiplegia. There was an earlier history of heart trouble and hypertension. He spoke rapidly and loudly, producing several stretches of fluent jargon (indicated below by the number of syllables), and paying little attention to many of the therapist's efforts to intervene. There were also major problems in his reading and writing. In this extract, the therapist is trying to establish whether the patient can identify various objects in the room.

T   'show me a pìcture/ on the wàll/
P   'picture on the wăll/ òh by (*2 syllables*)/ thère/ (*looks in wrong direction*) in the . (*2 syllables*) look at the er . whàt do they cáll them/ 'knights . of the chùrch/ and there (*1 syllable*) we can 'go no (*syllable*) and . of . over (*syllable*) . and (*2 syllables*) . there's pàrt of (*2 syllables*)
T   yès/ 'show me the pìcture/ of the mòuse/
P   the móuse/
T   'where's the pìcture/ of the mòuse/
P   òh/ 'picture of a môuse/ . pìcture/ . mòuse/
T   it's 'up on the wàll/ it's 'next to the càlendar/ . sée/ . hère/
P   thére/ . 'this one hère/
T   thàt one/
P   ôh/ . you've 'got to 'move ..
T   the 'calendar is 'next to thāt/ .
P   thàt's right/ . it's 'next to the 'person .
T   ÒK/
P   'that where . and 'there . and 'there something here as wèll/ somewhere 'other 'end of . (*4 syllables*) 'there's. . . .

In this sequence, the lack of comprehension is very much in evidence: the patient echoes the therapist's sentences, but does not relate them to the objects in question; several of his own sentences are unrelated to the theme being discussed; several are relatively 'empty' of meaning (e.g. *what do they call them*; *this one here*); several grammatical structures are begun, but they lead nowhere, and it is unclear what if any meaning they have for the patient. Overall, there is a confident, definite intonation, which in fact is no guide to the patient's ability. Once again, there is some blurring between the dysphasia categories, for there is also some suggestion of expressive (word-finding) problems, e.g. *look at the er*.

There are certain important issues in the aphasia literature which the above samples do not illustrate. The first concerns the extent to which all modalities of communication have been affected by the brain damage. The above discussion focuses on speech and listening comprehension; but what about reading and writing? Inability to read (*alexia*) and write (*agraphia*), along with their less severe forms (*dyslexia* and *dysgraphia*—though these terms are sometimes used to include the former, regardless of severity) may also be apparent, but in some patients reading and writing remains largely unaffected. It is also possible to have the one without the other (i.e. 'pure[16] alexia', or 'alexia without agraphia'), or to have the disorder focused *solely* on reading/writing ability, speech/auditory comprehension being largely unaffected. Because of the several possibilities for disturbance, full assessments of aphasia always include, as part of their battery of tests, components in which all four modalities of language are investigated. The theoretical significance of this point is considerable: if someone has completely lost the ability to speak and understand speech, for instance, but retains the ability to read and write, would it be reasonable to say that he has 'lost' language? Presumably not, as his reading/writing abilities evidently indicate that he can 'tap' a level of linguistic organization in his brain which remains undisturbed. Conversely, someone who was unable to use efficiently *any* of the four language modalities might provide evidence that the underlying language competence has been lost (at least in certain respects). This issue, as to whether aphasia is best seen as a fundamental disorder of the underlying linguistic competence all of us possess, or whether it is a more superficial disorder, affecting only aspects of our linguistic performance, is a currently controversial issue. Its resolution, of course, depends on many empirical studies of patients, for generalizations based upon only small samples (as has been the case so far) are inevitably misleading.

A second main issue concerns the extent to which the range of language's *uses* is affected in the various states of aphasia. In the above samples, we saw one use of language per patient. To what extent would the abilities represented there also turn up in other contexts of language use? The above samples were recorded in hospital clinics: would they also be representative of contexts outside (cf. p. 29)? Also, regardless of context, are there some kinds of language which the patient prefers to use? One category has often been recognized—the tendency of dysphasic patients to retain automatic, fixed phrases (such as *How do you do?*, *Fine thanks*) or serial sequences (such as counting, or reciting the days of the week). Even in very severe cases, it is common to find some of this sort of language frequently used, generally without comprehension. One patient, for example, had an excellent range of phrases for greeting and leave-taking, but little else.

A third big issue concerns the extent to which the notion of aphasia can be applied to children as well as adults. This is not a major problem if a stroke or other brain damage affects a young child, after he has acquired language: as with the adult, an aphasic condition can result.[17] But the term has also

---

[16] The term 'pure' is used to refer to a type of aphasia in which only one input or output modality is affected, i.e. speech *or* auditory comprehension *or* reading *or* writing.

[17] Even here, though, there are major differences. If the damage occurs sufficiently early on in the 'critical period' of language acquisition (cf. p. 51), some degree of spontaneous recovery will be apparent, and this will be very different in character, and much more rapid, than in the case of adults. The view is maintained that if the left hemisphere is extensively damaged, the right hemisphere is still sufficiently 'flexible' to be able to take over some of the functions of the left. See E. H. Lenneberg, *Biological foundations of language* (New York, Wiley 1967), Ch. 4.

been used to apply to children who, for some reason, have failed to develop language at all, or who have done so only partially or deviantly. The term *developmental aphasia/dysphasia* (sometimes, *childhood* or *infantile aphasia/dysphasia*) is often used in such cases, where the 'obvious' causes of undeveloped language can be ruled out (i.e. there is no evidence of deafness, mental retardation, motor disability, or severe emotional or personality problems). This is a kind of diagnosis by exclusion (cf. p. 20): in the absence of known alternatives, one concludes that there must be some minimal brain damage present, and it is this which justifies the extension of the term. Against this, it has been argued that, if aphasia means basically 'loss of language', then it is hardly right to use this label to apply to children who have not developed any language at all! Such children present very different problems of assessment and treatment—their difficulties are primarily educational, social and psychological, and not usually neurological. The point is a controversial one. The term is widely used in some parts of the world, and less so in others (including Great Britain). In this book, I shall not use it myself with reference to children, preferring to discuss child language delay and deviance as an independent category of disorder (see p. 160).

A further point is not to allow the broad distinctions in categories of aphasia to obscure the existence of quite specific syndromes which can be identified, affecting smaller groups of patients. For example, there is the syndrome called 'pure word deafness' (or sometimes, 'subcortical sensory aphasia'), a disorder which seems to affect auditory verbal recognition only, and which thus produces symptoms which resemble deafness. The patient will ask you to repeat words several times, for example, in an attempt to understand what you are saying. But he is not deaf: he can hear speech sounds in isolation, and can recognize the various noises of the environment. It is only when the speech sounds are combined into meaningful units that a problem arises; there is difficulty in recognizing what word it is that has been constructed; however, once recognized, there is no problem in comprehending it. Other aspects of language are unimpaired: the patient can express himself well, and has no problems with reading and writing. The suggestion is, therefore, that Wernicke's area is intact in such patients, but that there has been some damage to the pathways between this area and the auditory centres of the brain. Defined as such, it is a fairly rare disorder; it is much more likely that a patient will also have some degree of comprehension deficit. And as a second example of a more specific syndrome, there is the corresponding category of 'pure word blindness', in which the patient finds it difficult or impossible to interpret visually sequences of letters. He does not however have a problem if the words are spelt aloud, or even if they are drawn against the palm of his hand. The suggestion here is that there is damage to the visual cortex in the left hemisphere, and also to that part of the corpus callosum which transfers visual information from the right hemisphere.

It should be plain, both from the terminological confusion which exists within this subject, and also from the uncertainty with which different aphasic syndromes are postulated, that this is an area of language pathology which provides enormous scope for research—perhaps more than any other. There is a major need for detailed descriptive studies of aphasic behaviour, especially using the precise techniques of phonology, syntax and semantics (as outlined in Chapter 2). Very few detailed longitudinal studies have been carried out, and hardly any attempt has been made to correlate detailed linguistic descriptions with the patient's general medical progress, or the kind of therapeutic intervention he is receiving. There is doubt in the minds of some clinicians as to whether therapeutic intervention with many aphasic patients is worthwhile in the long term, given the amount of damage which has occurred, and the unlikelihood of making much progress, especially in a patient whose general faculties are in the process of deterioration anyway, on account of old age. But this is a premature conclusion, given that so little work has been done on evaluating strategies of linguistic intervention. The problem which has to be faced is how to get the research done, in a population like this one, where mortality is high and methodological problems abound. It may seem an easy matter to get together a group of aphasic patients for purposes of research; but in fact it is not. Obtaining a reasonably homogeneous group is not easy, in the first place. But even if obtained, the likelihood is that the majority of the group will either suffer further brain damage, other medical complications, or even die in the course of the study (see p. 194). It is a particularly intractable problem, and is the main reason why so much remains to be done.

But the importance of aphasia research is undenied—not only for clinical reasons (i.e. to help sufferers from the disorder) but also for theoretical reasons (to obtain a clearer understanding of the structure and function of the brain). Aphasia research has in fact been one of the main means of discovery about brain structure and function (cf. p. 91). This is the only syndrome where the various levels of language (grammar, vocabulary etc.) can be seen functioning separately from each other. By examining what can go wrong, and whereabouts in the language system that something goes wrong, suggestions can be made about 'how language works' which might be useful in other contexts than the clinical. Aphasia, it has been said (though not uncontroversially), is a key to our understanding of language as a whole.[18]

Agnosia, dyspraxia and dysarthria

Of special importance, in the differential diagnosis of linguistic pathology, is the need to distinguish aphasia from other categories of neurological

[18] A good place to start further reading in aphasia is with some of the early studies, such as the works by Henry Head (*Aphasia and kindred disorders of speech* (Cambridge, CUP 1926)) or the historical papers in Macdonald Critchley, *Aphasiology and other aspects of language* (London, Edward Arnold 1970). A classical text is by the Soviet psychologist, A. R. Luria, *Traumatic aphasia* (The Hague, Mouton 1970). A recent review, stressing the linguistic angle, is R. Lesser, *Linguistic investigations of aphasia* (London, Edward Arnold 1978).

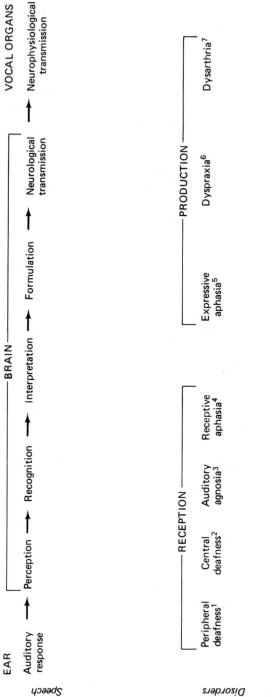

Fig. 36 The relationship of central language disorders to the communication chain
Notes: [1] see p. 133; [2] see p. 133; [3] see p. 151; [4] see p. 146; [5] see p. 143; [6] see p. 153; [7] see p. 155

etiology—in particular, from the notions of *agnosia* and *dyspraxia*. The basic situation, it will be recalled from Chapter 3, can be represented as in Figure 36. In a normal communication chain, the input side of speech involves four stages:

(a) response by the ear,
(b) perception by the brain,
(c) recognition by the brain,
(d) interpretation by the brain;

and on the output side, a further three stages:

(e) formulation of meaningful expression by the brain,
(f) controlled neurological transmission by the brain,
(g) controlled neurophysiological transmission by the vocal organs.

Each of these steps may be independently disordered, and the main associated terminology is introduced in Figure 36. These divisions are never as clearcut in reality as they are in theory; but let us begin, at least, with the essential theoretical claims being made by each of these categories.

We have already seen how perception of sound by the ear and the auditory centres of the brain can be interfered with at various points, and the clinical distinctions involved are classified as the main categories of deafness. But the fact that the brain perceives sound does not mean that it has the ability to *recognize* the sounds it perceives. The term *agnosia* is a general one, which is used whenever the brain apparently lacks the ability to recognize familiar objects, despite adequate sensory input. Any of the senses can be affected. Thus there is the phenomenon of *visual agnosia*—inability to identify visual stimuli; *tactile agnosia* (or *astereognosis*)—inability to identify objects by touch; and, in the same way, *auditory agnosia*. In this last category, a patient may have problems in identifying two instances of the same word, or sound, as being the same. Sounds that distinguish word meanings would be regularly confused. Sometimes, his actual ability to discriminate sounds might be affected; at other times, he can discriminate, i.e. say that the sounds are not the same, but be unable to see in what way they differ, and thus be unable to use this difference as part of the information he requires in order to understand speech. 'I can hear you talking, but I can't translate it,' said one such patient. The theoretical difference between this category and two others already referred to, *pure word deafness* and *Wernicke's aphasia* (or *auditory aphasia*) should be noted:

auditory agnosia: inability to recognize and differentiate sounds, words etc;
pure word deafness: ability to recognize sounds in isolation, but inability to integrate these into meaningful units; however, once decoded, comprehension is immediate; the syndrome is sometimes described as 'verbal' auditory agnosia;

Wernicke's aphasia: ability to recognize and integrate sounds, but inability to comprehend; speech, reading and writing usually affected.

However, as might be imagined, it becomes extremely difficult to 'see' these distinctions operating consistently in the behaviour of a patient. The evidence is often ambiguous. All we have to go on, after all, is the patient's response pattern to a stimulus. Take, for example, the following two situations. What evidence is there for a differential diagnosis, in terms of the above three distinctions?

1

T 'show me the tàble/
P oh yés/ tàble/ (*but not pointing at it*)
T yès/ the tàble/ where is it/
P 'one of those tàbles/ (*still not pointing*)
   well I sup'pose it 'might be (*looking around*) in a róom/
T yés/ (*encouragingly*)
P thère/ (*pointing to a chair*)

2

T 'show me the tàble/
P (*points, correctly*)
T now tèll me/ 'where's the tàble/
P (*looks uncertainly at her*)
T listen/ — 'where's the tàble/
P ta — ta —
T (*carefully*) tàble/ — tàble/
P 'ta-'ble/ òh/ tàble/ (*points, correctly*)

In the first extract, the evidence seems to support, fairly certainly, a diagnosis of Wernicke's aphasia. But the second case is more difficult. Is the patient's uncertainty because he is having difficulty in recognizing the constituent sounds of *table*, or is his problem one of being unable to integrate the sounds into a meaningful unit? Judging by the way he imitates the sounds quite well, and confidently points to the table once he has expressed the word himself, it would seem to be a case of pure word deafness—but what if his final decision had been a little less confident, or if he had made some errors in his attempt to imitate the word? We might then have felt that his difficulties were more fundamental.

Situations such as these are typical in clinical contexts. Of course, there are several strategies and tests available which can help to make a decision in such cases; but it would be wrong to leave the impression that it is always possible to sort out such cases. Indeed, diagnosis is often an uncertain and controversial matter.

A similar kind of ambiguity arises on the production side of the diagram. Let us assume a model of speech production in which the brain has 'decided' which meaning to convey, and has chosen a grammatical construction and the relevant vocabulary. All that remains is to give this abstract structure a phonological 'shape'. The evidence that a model of this kind has neurological reality comes from the disorder known as *apraxia*, or *dyspraxia*.[19] In its most general sense, apraxia refers to the disruption of the ability to produce a purposeful motor response; that is, the patient knows what he wants to do, but lacks control over the muscular activities required to perform a desired activity. Involuntary activities, however, using the same muscles, are not affected. So, for example, we might ask a patient to perform a particular motor task (such as to repeat the phrase *Good morning*), and he will be unable to do it. A little while later, however, we might notice that he had said the phrase automatically, while passing someone in the street. These difficulties in performing simple voluntary acts are by no means restricted to linguistic tasks, and indeed the neurological and neuropsychological classifications of apraxia are mainly concerned with nonlinguistic abilities. *Constructional apraxia*, for example, refers to a specific difficulty with visuospatial tasks, such as drawing, or arranging bricks in a certain order. In *apraxia for dressing*, the patient is unable to relate the forms of his clothes to that of his body. When speech is affected, the syndrome may be specified as *apraxia of speech, verbal* or *articulatory apraxia* (or *dyspraxia*): it then refers to a disruption in the ability to control the position of the muscles for speech, and the sequence in which they are used. Putting it briefly, the patient aims to say one sequence of sounds, and another comes out.

Here is an example of some adult dyspraxic speech. It is part of a conversation with a severely dyspraxic woman of 60, who had had a left CVA two years previously. It would seem from later in the extract that underlying the opening utterances is an attempt to produce the word *mill* or *milling*.[20]

T	you 'used to 'live on a fàrm/ dìdn't you/
P	yés/ yés/ . yés/
T	what 'sort of 'farm was thìs/
P	də . də . 'mɛnɛ . ədə . yes . there
T	did you have cóws on it/
P	yés/ . yés/ . də — əm — mɛ: . əm .
T	or 'was it cròps only/
P	yés/ . yés/ . əm . bə . pə . tʃ . ə:m — —
T	where wàs your 'farm/
P	jɛ — dɛ:
T	'was it around hére/
P	nó/ . nó/
T	'was it in Èngland/

[19] As with the aphasia/dysphasia distinction above, usage varies—*apraxia* implies a complete disruption of the motor activity involved; *dyspraxia* implies a partial disruption. Total disruption being uncommon, it is the latter term which is in general use in language pathology, for both the disorder and the patient (*dyspraxic*).

[20] It is difficult to be sure what the patient's target is, in spontaneous conversation of this kind. In order to analyse dyspraxic language, a structured test of articulation is always essential, in which the therapist knows in advance what word the patient is attempting to say.

P   tɪ . sjɔːs — də — təs . sɔːˈtə/
T   Yòrkshire/
P   yés/ yés/
T   ahà/ whereabòuts in ˈYorkshire/
P   əːm . əːm — ˈbɑːnz . tìn/
T   oh wèll/ gòod/ did you lìke it up ˈthere/
P   yês/ . yês/ . yês/
T   was it a bíg ˈfarm/
P   nó/ — there was — də — əːm . əːm — mənɪsp/ — òh/ whàt/ — — wɒˈrӕntən/ yès/ — əːm
T   can you wrìte it ˈfor me/
P   yès/ (*writes*) mìn/
T   a mìll/
P   yès/ yès/ . yès/ . yès/
T   I sèe/ — for pùmping/
P   nó/
T   was it for grìnding/
P   yés/ yés/ yés/
T   ˈgrinding whàt/
P   kɔːrs/
T   còrn/
P   yès/

Theoretically, the difference between dysphasia and dyspraxia is clear enough: it was neatly summarized by Henry Head in the following way: in the former, you cannot *say* what you want to; in the latter, you cannot *do* what you want to. But the important point is that the dyspraxic's inability to perform these motor movements is not due to any evident structural abnormality of the nervous system or in the muscles themselves. There is no paralysis, and little to go on by way of a clear sign that some deeprooted neurological problem is involved (there may, for example, be some associated difficulties with fine motor coordination). If an examination is made of the lips, tongue, palate, phonatory mechanism etc., everything seems normal. There is normal (or less disordered) use of language in other modalities, and normal awareness of vocabulary, grammar etc. within the speech modality. But as soon as the patient attempts to construct connected speech, other than for the most automatic of phrases, he encounters major difficulties of expression. His ability to repeat a sequence of the same sounds is also much reduced. The errors that are made are very inconsistent: a /p/ phoneme may emerge as a [p], [t], [f], etc. in a relatively short space of time; some sounds may perseverate (cf. p. 145) throughout a word or phrase, as in the following example from a dyspraxic child[21] of 4½, who had a tendency to perseverate on bilabials: *Christmas tree* was produced as /ˈpɪˈbɪˈpiː/ and /ˈbɪˈmɪˈpriː/; *elephant* as /hɛpɪpɪmp/. In the more severe cases, even vowels may be affected. Speech rhythm will tend to be slow and erratic, as the

[21] The theoretical problems over using such a phrase as 'developmental dyspraxia' are the same as those involved in the phrase 'developmental dysphasia' (cf. 148).

patient tries to obtain some measure of control. Difficulty in starting words may produce an effect which resembles stuttering (see p. 166).

This set of characteristics permits a potentially clear contrast to be made with aphasic symptomatology. The linguistic problems in dyspraxia are primarily identifiable at the phonological level, and do not affect other modalities; as a result, remediation involves a quite different kind of therapy. However, the fact that dyspraxia involves phonological as well as phonetic difficulties means that there must be some overlap with aphasia.

It is possible to make a theoretical distinction between dyspraxia and an expressive aphasia in which phonology has been affected (cf. p. 144): in the latter case, the phonological system itself is disordered (lacking the phonemes, or the correct rules governing their combination); in the former case, the phonological system is intact, but the patient is unable to control his use of it. It is somewhat like the difference between riding a bicycle with no handlebars, and one where the handlebars are present but not properly fixed to the frame, so that the bicycle does not respond to the rider. Unfortunately, the clinical situation is a fairly confused one, because (a) the term dyspraxia has sometimes been used to identify the phonological abnormalities of expressive aphasia, and (b) in many patients it is not clear whether the underlying system has been affected. There are several possible theoretical positions that may be taken up. For some, dyspraxia is a specific syndrome *within* expressive aphasia—just as specific as, say, word-finding or agrammatism (cf. above, p. 143). For others, it is felt that the qualitative differences between aphasia and apraxia are sufficiently great to warrant the two being seen as distinct syndromes, and this is the view represented above (Fig. 36). On this basis, we may have a patient displaying (a) dysphasic symptoms, with no dyspraxia (i.e. the phonological form of his limited expression of language is correct), (b) dyspraxic symptoms, with no dysphasia (i.e. his grammatical and semantic construction is correct (for his age), but his phonology is wrong), and (c) a mixture of both dyspraxia and dysphasia—which is perhaps the most common of the three possibilities, in adults. Category (b) is particularly common in children, involving a range of symptoms which may run from mild to severe.

This set of characteristics also permits a potentially clear contrast to be drawn with a further category of speech pathology, known as *dysarthria*. This is the name given to a series of motor speech disorders arising as a result of damage to the nervous system, and manifested by neuromuscular disability. Any aspect of speech production might be affected, depending on where in the central or peripheral nervous system the lesions occur; there may be problems of respiration, phonation, articulation or prosody; and other activities involving the vocal organs, such as chewing, swallowing, smiling, coughing, or sneezing may be affected. The term *anarthria* is not so widely used: it strictly means *total* inarticulateness due to neuromuscular insufficiency, and this is uncommon, compared with the varying degrees of partial insufficiency, ranging from mild to severe. Within this broad category, several specific syndromes have been established. *Ataxic*[22] *dysarthria*, for example, refers to the behavioural result of damage to the cerebellar system: it is characterized by a slowed, erratically-stressed utterance, with abnormally flat prosody, harsh voice quality, and considerable difficulty in articulation. Bilateral damage to the upper motor neurones can produce *spastic dysarthria*, a condition in which a limited and laboured range of muscular movement produces words with imprecise articulations, slurred sequencing, erratic pauses, flat prosody, and often accompanying facial grimaces. Other distinguishable types of dysarthria have been recognized, e.g. as a result of damage to the lower motor neurones, or to the extrapyramidal system.

In all these cases, however, there are several characteristics which make this disorder very different from dyspraxia. The most obvious difference is that the vocal tract muscles are plainly impaired in their movement (which is not the case with dyspraxia): a dysarthric patient might have considerable difficulty in moving his tongue around his mouth, whereas the dyspraxic's tongue would be quite mobile (though not necessarily under his control). There are clear signs of neurological insufficiency in this disorder, and often the dysarthria is simply one sign of a more general problem, such as cerebral palsy, or Parkinson's disease (identified in 1817 by the British surgeon, James Parkinson (1755–1824)), a degenerative disease of the basal ganglia, characterized by rigidity of muscles, a coarse tremor, and slowness and poverty of voluntary movement, with a typical mask-like face. The dysarthric usually has no difficulty in controlling his vocal organs, *within the limits of his muscular ability*; for instance, he will make respectable efforts to imitate words, when asked—unlike the dyspraxic, who will have great difficulty in organizing himself for this task. Again, unlike the dyspraxic, the articulatory and other errors will be fairly consistent, reflecting the fact that a single group of muscles is affected, and many of them will be outside the normal patterns of his language. If there is poor muscular control of the soft palate, for example, then abnormal nasalization will be a noticeable feature; if tongue movement is badly affected, vowels will be indistinct, and only rough approximations to many oral consonants will be heard; and so on. In short, the difference between dyspraxia and dysarthria is often very clear; but it must not be forgotten that the two types of production disorder can combine—the patient having problems both with his organizational ability for sounds and also with his ability to implement them. It will not always be obvious, without considerable investigation, which factor is predominant in accounting for a patient's difficulties with a particular type of sound.[23]

[22] *Ataxia* is a disorder characterized by tremors and a general lack of muscular coordination for both fine and gross motor activities.

[23] Further reading: Lord Brain, *Speech disorders: aphasia, apraxia and agnosia* (London, Butterworth, 2nd edn, 1965), J. W. Brown, *Aphasia, apraxia and agnosia* (Springfield, Ill., Thomas 1972), F. L. Darley, A. E. Aronson and J. R. Brown, *Motor speech disorders* (Philadelphia, Saunders 1975), R. Lesser, *Linguistic investigations of aphasia* (London, Edward Arnold 1978), Ch. 8.

Psychopathological language

Aphasia is the result of focal brain damage to the so-called 'language' centres. But what if the brain is damaged in other areas, or is subject to a general deterioration or change, in which the language centres are incidentally included? Or what if there is no detectable brain damage at all, and yet there is plainly some functional abnormality or inadequacy in behaviour, in which language, again, may be involved? We have seen how problems of this kind are grouped under the heading of psychopathology, the study of mental disturbance (cf. p. 67). Any of these may manifest itself in abnormal language—the language thus providing an important symptom of the disturbance, and often the only symptom. A person may begin speaking abnormally long before his disturbance affects other aspects of his behaviour. In psychotherapy, as we have seen, the entire focus of attention will be on the linguistic symptoms produced by the patient; and without these, it is impossible for treatment to proceed (if the patient does not talk to the psychiatrist, there is nothing the latter can do).

Perhaps because of the complexity of the conditions involved, the linguistic consequences of psychopathological disturbance have been more neglected than any of the other areas described in this book. Because of the influence of the medical model, attention has concentrated on those conditions where there is some tangible, physical evidence of disorder (*organic* conditions). The remainder have been consigned vaguely to some such label as *functional, psychogenic, nonorganic* (!), and so on. This distinction, as we have seen (p. 123) is often not very helpful in linguistic disability. More valuable would be detailed descriptive studies of the linguistic characteristics associated with the various psychopathological syndromes outlined in Chapter 3. For instance, several 'psycholinguistic' indices have been proposed as characteristic of schizophrenic behaviour: a narrowed and stereotyped vocabulary, often containing meaningless coinages (jargon), distorted phonology, idiosyncratic word associations, perseveration, inappropriate emotional expression (e.g. in intonation and tone of voice), sudden changes of direction in grammatical structure, incompleteness of structures, and a generally incoherent sequencing between sentences. Several of these features can be seen in the following sample, taken from a conversation with a female schizophrenic, in her mid-50s, with a long history of anxiety problems and institutionalization.[24]

```
T    you're in 'ward thirtèen now/
P    yès/
     yès/
     was —
     been —
     I've been —
     I'm — in — in —
     I'm in 'ward thirtèen/ .
```

[24] For transcription conventions, see p. 143.

T   how 'long have you been in 'ward thirtèen/
P   gòod 'while/
     a 'few 'years I thìnk/
     'two or three 'years I thìnk/
     I'm not —
     yès/
T   do you líke it on 'there/
P   not bád/ — ùsual/
T   have you 'got any frìends 'Mary/
P   from the sýna — er —
     'Anytown sỳnagogue/ .
     'please Gòd/ .
     I'll be gòing on the 'ninth of Jánuary/
T   you've got frìends 'there háve you/
P   yès/ .
     yès/ .
     fróm/ —
     'used to be with me ín/ —
     gòod while 'back/
     er — 'May in —
     'used to be 'with me gòod while 'back/
T   tèll me Máry/ . 'what 'things do you 'like dòing
P   I 'used to be 'in the 'laun —
     I was .
     I don't knów/
     they 'carried òn a bìt/ .
     but I 'don't knów/
     I mìght be going báck/ — —
     'Monday the sècond/ .
     I 'don't knów/ .
     it'll be 'bank hòliday hére/ .
     I 'don't knów/
     the fòllowing week/ —
     Sùnday/ —
     'Monday 'week I thìnk/

This patient would tend not to speak at all, unless directly questioned. Most of her sentences are short; many are unfinished; and there is much disjointedness between one sentence and the next. Her tendency to split up a meaning into smaller chunks, giving each a separate intonation unit, is clearly illustrated by the transcription, where the units are put on new lines. Her tendency to repeat, or partly repeat what she has said, is also noticeable. What does not appear in the transcript is an indication of her general behaviour throughout the conversation—in particular, the way in which she avoided eye contact, and generally left the therapist with no sense of 'rapport'. This is an important point, for without this impression of markedly asocial and eccentric behaviour, there are many features of the schizophrenic's language which might lead you to confuse it with aphasia.

There are reduced grammatical structures, jargon, perseveration and so on in both syndromes. Both types of patient may also be completely mute. But the differences usually resolve upon analysis: there is rarely a sense of a private barrier being erected between analyst and patient in aphasia; moreover, of course, the progress of schizophrenia can be controlled to some extent by drugs, which will produce dramatic changes in behaviour that would not be found in the slow progress made by the aphasic.

All aspects of language can have diagnostic or assessment value in psychopathology, and several specific measures have been proposed, apart from the above. If we measure the ratio of verbs to adjectives, or the proportions of different types of pronouns, for example, it is possible to show some interesting correlations. The whole range of prosodic features of the voice is of major significance, especially in such a syndrome as manic depression (cf. p. 69). We can investigate the failure to achieve satisfactory sequencing of ideas or syntax, both in the patient's own monologue, and also in his dialogue with others. A common indication that something is psychologically wrong (common, for example, in children diagnosed as autistic)[25] is the tendency for the patient not to respond directly to conversational stimuli, but to keep up a monologue of his own, as the following extract illustrates:

T   'what are you going to 'do with 'that car nòw/
P   I like my cár/ (*pushing it on floor*)
T   lòok/ . I've got 'one like thát/
P   in hère it 'goes/ (*pushing car into garage*)
T   'don't for'get to 'shut the dóors/
P   'find the màn nów/ (*looking about*) . . .

In each case the child ignored, or seemed to ignore, the therapist's stimulus sentence, and yet by keeping up a flow of language an 'apparent' conversation was obtained.

It is impossible to generalize about language in the context of mental retardation. There is no straightforward correlation between any of the many syndromes and the language produced. A group of Downs' syndrome patients, for example (cf. p. 21) will produce a wide range of individual differences in their linguistic capabilities. Perhaps the only safe claim that can be made is that when subnormality becomes really severe,[26] there will be

---

[25] *Autism* is the name given to a complex pattern of abnormal behaviour, especially identifiable in early childhood, in which there are bizarre interpersonal relationships (such as avoidance of eye contact, lack of response to others, no attempt to initiate contacts, preference for objects rather than people), obsessive concern with sameness in the environment, and with repetitive activities, and little or no attempt to intitiate and respond to communication. See further D. J. Cohen & A. M. Donnellan (eds), *Handbook of autism and pervasive developmental disorders* (Chichester, Wiley 1987).

[26] This is not the place to go into the many approaches which have been developed to assess levels of mental retardation in children. In Britain, since the Education (Handicapped Children) Act of 1970, a distinction has been drawn between severe and moderate levels of educational subnormality (ESN(S) and ESN(M) respectively), the distinction being based on intelligence, as measured by certain tests. New proposals for all categories of special education in Britain (i.e. including the blind, deaf, physically handicapped, maladjusted, etc.) emerged in 1978 in the Warnock Report: *Special educational needs*

no language—which is hardly a brilliant insight. And yet, even here there is great scope for research. Even in the minimally purposive behaviour of the most severely handicapped, there may be signs of pattern, or desire to communicate, which might be made the basis of a teaching programme. What upon first encounter might seem to be random grunts may on analysis turn out to be a systematic use of a very limited vocal apparatus. Everything depends, it would seem, on the investigator and teacher finding the right mode of input to the child, and to *keep* trying, if early attempts to make contact fail. It is an easy, and a natural reaction, to give up with such children, and conclude that 'he just won't learn'. Such comments, properly interpreted, can only mean: 'so far, I have not been able to find a way to enable him to learn.' Whether it is practical or economical to keep trying, of course, given the pressing demands of others for attention, is a difficult and often emotional decision. But theoretically, at least, the answer is plain: of course one keeps trying. And from the analytical point of view what this means, usually, is careful analysis—not only of the language of the child (if any) but of the language of his environment, from which he is attempting to learn. How carefully has this been structured, to enable him to make best sense of it? One of the general problems with mentally retarded children or adults is the problems they have in resolving a large number of competing stimuli. They cannot cope with too many inputs at once, but get confused. Using this guideline, then, we can look at the language inputs to the child, to see whether they are too complex for him. It is very easy for complexity to creep in, unnoticed. One child's small teddy was being referred to as 'teddy', 'cuddly', 'Fred', and other names, by the people who came into contact with him; no-one had bothered to check whether they were all using the same language to the child, and as a result unwittingly complicated his world, in this small but crucial respect. Standardizing the learning environment, and yet not making it so stereotyped that there is no potential for growth and creativity: this is one of the main methodological issues facing those who work in mental retardation.[27]

Developmental language disorders
Most of the children who are noticeably behind their chronological peers in their ability to produce or comprehend speech fall into one of two categories: they are mentally retarded, to some degree; or they suffer from a degree of hearing loss. A significant number of children, however, manifest

(HMSO), in which the major recommendation was made that 'the term "children with learning difficulties" should be used in future to describe both those children who are currently categorized as educationally subnormal and those with educational difficulties who are often at present the concern of remedial services' (43)—these difficulties being then graded as mild, moderate or severe, with the label 'specific' being used in cases where the learning difficulty is restricted to a particular problem (such as reading). This nomenclature, it is argued, gives a better indication of the child's disabilities, and is less likely to stigmatize the child (as such labels as 'severely subnormal' did).

[27] For a review of the field, see Harold Vetter, *Language behavior and psychopathology* (Chicago, Rand McNally 1969); on mental handicap in particular, see A. F. Ashman & R. S. Laura (eds), *Education and training of the mentally retarded: recent advances* (London, Croom Helm 1985).

neither of these problems, and yet are still well behind their peers in language ability. These are the children who have been referred to as 'developmentally dysphasic', but their diagnosis is classically one of exclusion (cf. p. 20): there is no deafness, no psychiatric difficulty (such as retardation, maladjustment, or severe emotional problems), and no evident neurological damage. On the other hand, they do display psychological, social and educational problems—though whether these are the cause or the result of the linguistic difficulty remains an imponderable.

The influence of the way adult brain disorders have been investigated has been strong on this field. Neurological hypotheses have been advanced, referring to 'minimal brain damage' or to a delay in neurological maturation. The motor/sensory distinction has also been invoked, so that such children are regularly referred to as 'expressive' or 'expressive-receptive' (or, on occasion, 'receptive', though convincing examples of a purely receptively disordered child—analogous to a Wernicke's aphasic, cf. p. 146—are not easy to find).[28] The difficulty with this approach is that it is not so easy to apply in the case of children: putative syndromes of developmental disorder are rarely as clear as those advanced for adult disorders; and few children come to autopsy, so that neurological hypotheses can be checked.

In recent years, however, a great deal of progress has been made in our understanding of the bases of these disorders, through a range of psychological and linguistic studies which have investigated the problem from several interrelated points of view. Two broad hypotheses have been advanced: firstly, that the disorders are a consequence of a more fundamental deficit of a psychological nature; secondly, that the disorders are a result of damage to the linguistic processing system alone. There is evidence to suggest that both hypotheses are right, some of the time. There is clear evidence that some of these children have deficits in their auditory perception ability (cf. p. 119); some have problems in their auditory storage capacity (a very poor auditory short-term memory, for instance—cf. p. 63); some have difficulty in processing the information perceived through the auditory channel (requiring slowly-presented inputs); and some have difficulty in attending to sequences of items presented auditorily (a 'reduced auditory attention span'). An interesting feature is that the rhythmical abilities of many of these children are poor, both in nonverbal as well as prosodic ways (e.g. in dancing, movement, or tapping rhythms out). Some have poor awareness of symbolic behaviour generally, showing poor appreciation of what is involved in play, or gesture (particularly the case with children displaying autistic tendencies, cf. p. 159). Some are highly distractible and disorganized in all aspects of their behaviour (*hyperkinetic* or *hyperactive* children). All of this adds up to a view that many of these children have definite cognitive problems, especially in relation to auditory

---

[28] In early studies, this second category was referred to as 'congenital word deafness' or 'congenital auditory imperception': cf. p. 133 above.

imperception and attention control. If they do have these problems, then naturally their speech processing abilities will be affected. The disorder is not primarily one of speech structuring in the brain, on this view; and treatment would proceed primarily on the basis of attacking the underlying cognitive difficulty, e.g. by working on attention, space/time relationships, symbolic play or rhythmic skills.

By contrast, there are several children (as many as a third, according to some estimates) who display the same kind of marked language delay, but who seem to have few difficulties with any of the tasks referred to in the previous paragraph. On general sensory processing and auditory processing tasks, their performance is within normal limits, or only slightly abnormal. The analysis of their language brings to light a range of abnormal patterns which it is difficult to associate with any psychological explanation, and we are forced to conclude that the problem is restricted to the linguistic processing system as such. These difficulties may be purely phonetic, affecting solely the articulatory musculature, in which case we could talk about a *developmental dysarthria*, purely and simply; or, the difficulties might be primarily phonological, in which case the most relevant term to use would be *developmental dyspraxia* (cf. p. 154). The term *developmental dysphasia* might then be reserved (if it were used at all) for those developmental disorders in grammar and semantics, insofar as the primary manifestation of the disorder was identifiable in linguistic terms. An important piece of evidence here would be the extent to which the disorder manifests itself in other modes than speech in the written language of those who have been taught to write. It is too early to be certain, but preliminary studies have shown some systematic abnormalities in the written language of children classed as dysphasic, and these features seem to be very different from those encountered in other categories of pathology (e.g. in the written language of deaf children).

Here is an example of a child who was diagnosed as having an expressive language problem. His comprehension of speech, using one of the standard tests, was normal for his age; hearing was within normal limits—indeed, everything that could be tested was within normal limits. The only trouble was that he was producing language such as the following, and he was four years of age:

T   nòw/ 'here's the bóok/ — 'this is the 'book we were 'looking at befòre/ isn't it/
P   tèddy bear/
T   there's a tèddy bear/ yès/
P   'teddy a hòme/
T   you've 'got one at hŏme/
P   yèah/
T   'what do you càll him/ — —
P   a tèddy bear/
T   has he 'got a náme/
P   yèah/ — he nàme/

T   what is it/
P   er
T   'what's his nàme/ —
P   tèddy bear/
T   tèddy bear/
P   yèah/
T   does he — do you 'keep him in your bédroom/
P   yèah/ —
T   whère in your 'bedroom does he 'live/
P   don't knòw/
T   you don't knòw/ — — 'let's have a 'look at these pìctures/ — 'what's thàt/
P   a bàth/
T   yès/ — and 'what's thàt/
P   dùck/
T   yès/ — there's anòther 'duck like thát one/
P   sàme/
T   sàme/ 'that's rìght/ 'good bòy/ — and 'what's thàt/ — — — do you knów/
    (*points to towel in the picture*)
P   swìmming/ —
T   it's a tòwel/
P   tòwel/
T   that's rìght/ yès/ — I 'wonder who's 'going to gò in that 'bath/
P   mè/

Three kinds of information are necessary before we can carry out a linguistic assessment of children with developmental language disorders. First, we must have descriptive information, so as to be able to identify and label every feature of the language being used or responded to by the patient. This will basically take the form of a phonological and a grammatical description (see Chapter 2). What we must remember is that to be really useful the description must be systematic and comprehensive: it is not enough to collect a few examples of abnormal structures or sounds that happen to have caught your attention. Only a systematic description, supported if necessary by statistical analysis, can provide a solid foundation for assessment conclusions to be drawn. Secondly, we need information about the strategies of linguistic interaction being used between therapist and child: what means are being used to elicit language, and how far does the child himself initiate conversation? Is the child being involved in a free-moving conversation, or are his tasks being linguistically structured in some way (for example, is he being asked to imitate, to complete a sentence, to choose between alternatives)? Differences in the sampling situation, and in task difficulty, need to be carefully watched in carrying out assessment (cf. p. 29). Thirdly, it is necessary to grade the sounds and structures encountered, in order to provide a yardstick for carrying out assessment and treatment. It is this last point on which most attention has been focused. The usual (some would say the only) way of grading linguistic features is to arrange them in terms of their expected order of appearance as found in studies of normal language acquisition (cf. p. 52). Scales of language acquisition are established, on which are placed in sequence those sounds/structures which appear first in normal children, which appear next, and so on. Not everything is known about the acquisition of language, of course, and so there will be many gaps in these scales, but enough information is these days available to enable the task to be carried out, at least in outline, in the form of general assessments and profiles of individual children. The following sentences illustrate some aspects of this developmental progress in the area of grammar: on the left is an indication of age; on the right are given some sentences that might be expected to be in use at that time:

16 months	dàddyʃ gòne/ mòre/ thère/ nò/ tèddy/
21 months	'daddy thère/ 'see dàddy/ 'want bòok/ nò 'potty/ 'big càr/ 'in bòx/ whère téddy/
24 months	'want that càr/ my dàddy 'gone/ bòx in thére/
27 months	'daddy 'kick bàll/ 'teddy gòne nów/ 'where 'that tèddy 'gone/ 'want more mìlk in thére/
30 months	'daddy gone 'town in càr/ 'me 'want mòre thóse/ that 'man do 'kick that bàll/ 'where you 'put that 'big càr/
36 months	'daddy 'gone in the gàrden/ and he did 'fall òver/ you 'pick that bàll up/ 'cos it's prètty/

Even if no further information is given about the types of structures that characterize each age range, it should now be possible to make informed guesses about the likely level of developmental delay involved in the child illustrated above—or with the following set of sentences, taken from a conversation with another 4-year-old:

the 'cat had kìtten/	'Mummy 'house 'be in thère/
it blàck/	it 'have a 'nice bèd/
yès/	'what it 'doing nòw/
it 'play 'lots and lòts/	it 'fall òver/[29]
'mother cat lìke it/	
it crỳing/	

A similar kind of progression could be established for the development of phonology (see further, p. 180).

No mention has so far been made of semantic development. Undoubtedly, the more we learn about the normal processes of semantic development in children, the more we will be able to understand what is taking place in developmental disorders. But, as pointed out in Chapter 2 (p. 45), work in semantics lags far behind the other domains. All I can do in this book is express caution about the use of oversimplified measures, such as the idea of vocabulary counting. It would seem to be an obvious thing to do—to estimate a child's developing linguistic capacity by working out the size of his vocabulary—and estimates are often given, for children at different ages. The trouble is that these estimates vary enormously. One pair of estimates for 5-year-olds varied from 2000 words to 10,000 words. Why is

[29] Most of these sentences have three main clause elements, but there is plainly some uncertainty, especially about verbs. In terms of the above progression, a level of 24–27 months is suggested.

this? One reason is the difficulty in identifying what is to count as a word in spoken language (cf. *it's, shan't*, etc.—one word or two?). Another is that everything depends on what kind of vocabulary we are thinking of: is it *active* vocabulary (i.e. words the child actively uses) or *passive* vocabulary (i.e. words the child knows, but does not himself use)? The latter will be a much larger figure. Then there is the problem of how to be sure that the child does indeed *know* the vocabulary we are counting. A child who uses such words as *reptile* or *dinosaur* may be getting them only half right—as one child did who pointed at a picture of tyrannosaurus rex and called it a lion. The problem for the vocabulary counter is this: does he include this word in his estimates of that child's knowledge, or exclude it? There are arguments both ways. Lastly, there is the problem of different senses of the same word: should we count *top* (meaning summit) and *top* (meaning toy) as the same or different words? If that seems an easy decision, then what about the twenty or so meanings of most of the common verbs in the language—*take, give, get* etc.? It is for such reasons that vocabulary development is a field which it is difficult to make firm decisions about, and thus difficult to use in clinical language studies. We can make rough estimates, but little more. Of far greater importance is to see how the vocabulary is used by the child—or, in other words, how the child puts his vocabulary into sentences and differing situations (which is what a grammatical analysis is basically trying to do).

Lastly, in this connection, we should recall the danger of introducing classifications into this field which may be misleading in their apparent simplicity. Two such classifications were mentioned in the introduction to this chapter: the delay/deviance distinction, and the organic/functional distinction. The first is potentially valuable, insofar as it is supplemented by more detailed descriptive studies. The second is of limited value, for by definition all the disorders in this section are 'functional', and yet they are plainly of several different types. The point is worth mentioning, as it is fairly common to see these disorders prefixed by the term 'functional', e.g. 'functional articulation disorder', to refer to a developmental disability in phonology which is not explicable with reference to the usual range of organic criteria. In this case, as there is a clear contrast evidenced between this kind of articulation problem and that where there is clear sign of organic damage, as in developmental dysarthria, the usage may be helpful. By the same token, the absence of any clearly distinct syndromes under the headings of grammar and semantics suggests that it would be of little value to apply the term in such contexts: labels such as 'functional grammatical disorder' or 'functional language disability' should therefore be avoided.[30]

---

[30] A review of research in this field is M. A. Wyke (ed.), *Developmental dysphasia* (London, Academic Press 1978). A linguistic emphasis is illustrated in D. Crystal, P. Fletcher and M. Garman, *The grammatical analysis of language disability* (London, Cole & Whurr, 2nd edn. 1988). A widely used (in Great Britain) intervention programme based on psychological principles is introduced in J. Cooper, J. Reynell and M. Moodley, *Helping language development* (London, Edward Arnold 1978). The multidisciplinary approach to the problem is well illustrated in W. Yule & M. Rutter (eds), *Language development and disorders* (London, Mac Keith Press 1987).

Pathologies of production

In our model of speech production, a general distinction was made between the formulation of meaningful expressions and their organization in phonological terms, on the one hand, and the subsequent encoding and transmission of these linguistic units through the neurological-physiological-anatomical pathways, to give these units phonetic reality, on the other. Disorders of the first type were discussed under the headings of either aphasia or dyspraxia. It remains now to consider the range of disorders which interfere with the process of phonetic encoding. There are three types of interference recognized in the speech pathology literature:

(a) interference with the sequencing of linguistic units in connected speech; this raises problems of *fluency*;

(b) phonetic interference with the source of phonation which will 'carry' the linguistic message; this raises problems of *voice*;

(c) interference with the phonetic realization of the abstract units that constitute the linguistic system; this raises problems of *articulation*.

We have already had cause to discuss one of the types of articulation disorder—dysarthria—in the context of our discussion of apraxia. But what sort of thing is involved under the other headings?

Disorders of fluency

The popular sense of fluency refers to the degree of proficiency someone has developed in performing a motor activity. In relation to language, the term implies ease and rapidity of speaking, a continuous flow with little hesitation, and a good command of grammar and vocabulary. In speech pathology, these implications are also present, but when the notion of *nonfluency* is discussed, it is usually with reference to specific disturbances in the rhythm and timing of speech, and not to such notions as size of vocabulary. The terms *arhythmia* and *dysrhythmia* are sometimes used to refer to phonetic interference with the normal rhythms of speech—one might be 'mildly' or 'severely' dysrhythmic, for instance, or (wholly) arhythmic. But the usual terms to describe the main nonfluency syndromes are *stuttering*[31] and *cluttering*; and it is in relation to the first of these that most investigation has been carried out.

Stuttering seems a very obvious category of speech disorder; but it is in fact one of the most complex to describe and define precisely. The trouble is (as we have seen elsewhere in this book) that stutterers are hardly ever exactly alike. It is as if there is a pool of characteristics of disfluent speech, and any one stutterer picks out of this pool some of these characteristics. These characteristics can be grouped into seven main types:

1 An abnormal amount of segment, syllable, word or phrase *repetition*, as in *p-p-p-- please, the pol- pol- policeman, I think he's got a — got a — got a—* .

---

[31] The term stammering is also used, especially in Great Britain, to refer to exactly the same set of behaviours.

2 Obstructions to the air-flow, due to the inability to release the tension that has built up in preparing to articulate a sound: on a tape, the result is a long pause; but face to face there may be many signs of the struggle that is going on within for control—facial spasms and grimaces, sudden movements of the head, or of the whole body, and awkward gestures. This phenomenon is referred to as *blocking*, and the individual sounds affected as *blocks* or *hard contacts*.

3 Abnormal prolongations of sound segments, as in *f-f-f-feels*, where the initial *f* is being produced as a single lengthened sound, and not with brief pauses between (cf. (1) above).

4 The introduction of extra words or sounds with a solely emotional force at points of difficulty, e.g. *gosh, oh, tut*.

5 Erratic stress patterns in words, and abnormal intonation and tempo patterns on sentences, mainly because of the very hesitant speech, and the accompanying irregular breathing.

6 Words being left unfinished.

7 Awkward circumlocutions: the stutterer may know very well which types of sound cause him particular problems, and will therefore go out of his way (linguistically) to avoid saying them—sometimes to quite surprising lengths: one stutterer, in the middle of a story, said '. . . and lying in the road was one of those—animals that meow. . .'.

To illustrate some of the effects encountered in stuttering, here is an extract from a conversation with a fairly severe adult male stutterer:[32]

T   and do you 'have any hòbbies/
P   yès/ — òne . 'of — my . 'hob — — bies/ . is 'mus — sìc/ . and the óther — —
     'one/ is erm — 'playing — — hòckey/ — —
T   'when you say músic/ do you 'mean do you 'like listening tó it/ or 'do you plày
     'anything/
P   I — — I 'actually — — plày in/ — — 'two erm — bànds/ 'and 'I 'als . so . 'like
     lìst . e . ning — — to 'mus . 'sic/ — —
T   'what do you plày/
P   I — — erm — well — — my — —
T   I 'mean what ìnstrument/
P   yès/ quìte/ — — 'my máin 'instru — ment is the/ — erm — (h h) is the — —
     'bass . gui — tàr/ — — but 'I 'also 'play — — the erm bán — — jo/ and
     òrdinary — gui — 'tar/

This extract shows the way the 'transition smoothness' between sounds, syllables, words, phrases and larger units can be interfered with. Nonfluency, it should be plain, is a much larger phenomenon than is suggested by the traditional view—that stutterers have problems with sounds. It is *not* just a matter of sounds: it is a problem of the entire rhythmic

---

[32] These excerpts are based on transcripts in P. Dalton and W. J. Hardcastle, *Disorders of fluency* (London, Cole & Whurr, 2nd edn. 1988). Several phonetic details have been omitted, e.g. the first occurrence of *guitar* was pronounced /skwiːʔ—taː/, *and* was pronounced /ən/, *the erm* was pronounced /ðəm/.

organization of speech, suggestive of a deeprooted neurological problem affecting that part of the brain which controls the timing and sequencing of speech patterns. But we are nowhere near identifying this 'explanation' in neurological terms.

There is a second reason why a watertight definition of stuttering is so difficult to achieve, and that is the problem of distinguishing it from what is called *normal nonfluency*. For example, it is perfectly normal to hesitate in our speech: indeed, it has been estimated that two-thirds of our spoken language comes out in chunks of six words or less. About 30 per cent of an average conversation consists of—silence. And if we listen carefully to an ongoing conversation, we will be able to hear other nonfluencies also— changes of direction in mid-sentence, prolongations of sounds, and several types of sound or syllable repetition. Some clinicians have in fact argued, on the basis of this, that *no* boundary line can be drawn between stuttering and normal speech. Nor is it simply a matter of degree, with a single continuum from the one state to the other: some experiments have shown that at certain linguistic tasks (such as word repetition in controlled settings) there is always a proportion of stutterers who are in fact *more* fluent than the population of non-stutterers brought in as controls! On the other hand, it is not the case that the frequency of these errors, taken all together, is to be found in normal speech, and there are certain characteristics of stuttering which are hardly ever to be found there—the blocking phenomenon being a case in point.

The distinction becomes particularly sensitive when we observe young children, at certain points in their speech development. It has been said that 'all kids stutter'—by which is meant that young children (say, between two and five) have an abnormally high amount of word repetition in their speech, compared with adults, and from time to time become noticeably nonfluent in their production of initial segments too. Take the following extract from a three-year-old:

> and — and — my 'daddy did — did 'fall off the làdder/ and he — he — he — did 'hurted his knèe/ and it was — it was 'all sòre . . .

While this might sound like stuttering—and many parents do indeed refer to it as such—it can be argued that it should not really be interpreted in this way, as the nonfluency is probably only a consequence of the language acquisition process. Any of us might well begin to stutter in a novel or exciting language-using situation, and for the child to be doing this in the middle of his language learning period, it might be argued, is only natural, and not, accordingly, something that should be pejoratively labelled as a 'stutter' (nor, of course, to be picked upon and 'corrected').[33]

A further problem about the definition of stuttering is that it needs to take

[33] Indeed, it has been argued that parents who do this are possibly laying the foundations for a more serious stuttering problem later on; drawing the child's attention to it and calling it a mistake must surely threaten the child's confidence in his own language-using ability.

into account the *context* in which the stutter appears. From casual acquaintance, we might well think that stutterers stutter consistently, but this is not usually the case. One clinic uses a questionnaire which they ask all stutterers to fill in when they first attend. It includes such questions as: 'Under what conditions is your stammer most severe? Under what conditions is your speech most fluent? Do you try to avoid any particular speech situations (e.g. shopping)?' Another scale, which attempts to evaluate the patient's attitudes towards his stutter, asks him to make true/false judgements about himself with reference to such statements as:

I find it easy to talk with almost anyone
A person who is my teacher or my boss is hard to talk to
I often ask questions in group discussions
I dislike introducing one person to another

These questions illustrate the general point: stuttering varies enormously from person to person, and from situation to situation. The clinician's aim, accordingly, is to establish those situations which cause the stutterer most anxiety, and to devise treatment programmes which will enable him to begin to cope with such situations.

It is when we investigate the attitudes of stutterers towards their own communicative abilities, and towards their stutter in particular, that we encounter a peculiar problem: how they rate their fluency may be quite different from how it is rated by other people. You may be struck by someone's stutter, and may have some mild difficulty in attending to him (until you adapt), but you may not feel that his problem is particularly serious, and you may actually say this to him (if, for instance, he apologized for his stutter). But this attitude of the listener is probably vastly different from the feelings the stutterer privately holds about his inarticulateness. At one London clinic, a group of adult stutterers were asked about their feelings about their own stutters.[34] Many of them were greatly preoccupied with their speech, whatever the level of severity of their stutter. Some of them were very anxious about it; others were simply alert to the prospective difficulties involved in speaking—always scanning ahead to see if any problem words were coming up. An interesting consequence of this is that several said they thought this made them poor *listeners*, because they were concentrating too much on what they themselves were saying. Many of the more severe cases complained of the amount of physical and mental energy taken up by this activity, amounting at times to exhaustion.

Several spoke of cutting down any explanation needed to the bare minimum, simplifying an argument to the points they felt they could make easily. Some gave up argument altogether, agreeing with another speaker rather than getting involved in complicated disagreement. Others even spoke of saying the opposite of what they felt, because it happened to be easier. . . .
The therapists were under the impression for several weeks that a member of the

[34] This account is given in P. Dalton and W. J. Hardcastle, *op. cit.*, 97–9.

group was engaged to be married, because, when asked if he was married he replied, 'Pending'. What he meant to say was that he was divorced, but he was having great trouble with 'd' at that time. (Dalton and Hardcastle, *op. cit.*, 98)

Such accounts are most illuminating in providing the non-stutterer with a sense of the nature of the problem, and illustrate also a major task for the therapist: before she can make progress, she must develop in the stutterer a more realistic sense of his communicative strengths and weaknesses, getting him to see how much of his problem is the outcome of his own strategies for coping, which in some cases might have hindered rather than helped.

Research into stuttering is complicated, then, by the need to keep both structural and situational variables in mind. Not only is it important to have a precise understanding of the linguistic basis of the difficulty (i.e. a clear description of the linguistic contexts in which the breakdowns in transition smoothness occur), but we must also have as full an understanding as is possible of the psychological and social factors which contribute to the difficulty. Only then is a systematic treatment rationale possible. There are many classifications and theories of stuttering behaviour, and one reason for their number, and for the controversy that exists within the literature on stuttering, is the different emphases that clinicians place on these variables, and the relationships between them. For example, an early classification of stuttering into two broad types relies very much on the importance of the psychological factors involved. *Primary* stuttering is seen as an episodic stutter in which there is no anxiety, struggle or self-awareness on the part of the stutterer; there would be no defensive reactions about his stutter, and indeed he may not even refer to his speech difficulties as such. A gradient of increasing severity is then postulated, with the stutter becoming more chronic and the person more self-aware (*transitional* stuttering), until the phenomenon could be called *secondary* stuttering. In this condition there is full awareness (real or imagined) of the existence of the problem, and major attempts are made to modify or avoid the stutter, leading to the uncontrolled, tense and irregular characteristics of speech referred to above. These distinctions are often referred to by clinicians, but it is doubtful if they have any theoretical value, given the range of variables which are subsumed under each heading. And many clinicians deny that the first category should be called a type of stuttering at all; for them, the role of the avoidance reaction is crucial.

Major disagreements also abound over the main theoretical question: what is the cause of a stutter. The short answer is easy, but unilluminating: there is no single cause. As a long answer, we could commence a survey of the several dozen proposals that have been seriously developed; but it will perhaps suffice for the present book to refer only to the main lines of thinking. In this way, the proposals may be grouped into four broad types.

1 There are several *organic* theories of stuttering, in the sense that the individual is said to have a genetic or physical predisposition to stutter which

is 'released' when environmental stress becomes great. One view tries to relate stuttering to neurological problems which arise as the result of mixed cerebral dominance: because the two hemispheres are 'competing' for dominance, interference in the natural process of neurological encoding takes place, and the result is manifested as a stutter. An alternative neurological theory proposes a defect in brain structure so that there is a predisposition to perseverate when using language, with the result being a stutter. Biochemical reasons have also been advanced: a chemical imbalance which interferes with the way impulses are transmitted along neurones or across synapses (such as a defect in myelination). And a further theory argues that there must be defects in the auditory feedback mechanism between vocal organs, ear and brain (cf. p. 58), so that the individual becomes unable to monitor his output efficiently, and stuttering is the result.

2 There are several *psychoneurotic* theories of stuttering, which attempt to relate stuttering to factors in the personality of the stutterer, or in his emotional relationship with the environment. One group of theories tries to identify personality types as stutterers—perhaps over-anxious or over-hostile individuals. In its extreme form, it is suggested that the denial of basic psychological needs as a child has formed the stuttering personality (a view based on Freudian theory (cf. p. 70)). Inadequate contact with the mother (e.g. while suckling) or overprotection have been advanced as possible causes. Disturbed interpersonal relationships, from whatever underlying cause, could also be involved.

3 Overlapping with (2), there are several *anxiety* theories of stuttering. Stuttering is felt to begin because the speaker believes that speech is a problem, that he has failed, or will fail. He may have been told this directly, as when children are prematurely corrected by their parents for normal nonfluency (cf. above): the feelings of impatience generated by anxious parents who disapprove of nonfluency produce insecurity and anxiety in the child, and a worsening of the behaviour. This 'diagnosogenic' theory is well summarized by one of its main proponents, the American speech pathologist Wendell Johnson, who argues that stuttering begins not in the child's mouth, but in the listener's ear! Sometimes a more indirect process of development takes place, the child perceiving the adverse reactions of listeners to his own 'primary' stutter (cf. above), and gradually developing a tendency to avoid and fear certain linguistic situations which cause him difficulty, which in turn promotes the stutter.

4 Overlapping with (3), there are also several theories of stuttering based on *learning* theory, i.e. those studies which try to establish how learning takes place in an individual, by identifying the factors which promote motivation, the nature of successful stimuli, and the kind of reinforcement which is needed to maintain the learned behaviour. One view, for example, maintains that stuttering is the result of an inner conflict: should one speak or not speak, make contact with another person or not make contact (an 'approach-avoidance' view). Another view argues that stuttering occurs in

situations which have unpleasant associations for the speaker, i.e. he has developed a negative emotional response to these situations, and this manifests itself in stuttering.

Typologies of this kind inevitably run into difficulties, however. There is evidently a great deal of overlap between the categories, because of the close interdependence of the factors upon each other. And it is this which makes any single theory of stuttering unlikely to be agreed. Personality, situation, genetic predisposition, social interaction and cultural expectation are inevitably closely linked. Different types of stutterer will doubtless emerge as the result of different combinations of factors. The multiple origins of stuttering in a group, and even within an individual, is a safer view to adopt than to go for one or other of the above theories. It is, moreover, often difficult to decide between the competing claims of the various theories, because there is insufficient evidence. How would you go about obtaining evidence to support your view that an adult stutterer had had his stutter misdiagnosed by his parents when he was three? Case histories of stutterers invariably ask questions about the person's early life, for example:

Did your stutter handicap you at school?
Did you regard your parents as lenient or strict in their discipline?
What do you consider to be your most vivid and unpleasant memory associated with stuttering?

But a complete or wholly accurate picture is obviously going to be impossible to obtain. Or again, to take another theory, how would you decide if the anxiety and hostility of the patient in your clinic was the cause of the stutter (cf. (2) above) or the result of the stutter (cf. (4) above)? There is a 'chicken and egg' aspect to this problem—the anxiety feeds the stutter which feeds the anxiety which . . . or did the stutter come first?

The need for accurate assessment is crucial, if anything more than the briefest success is to be obtained in therapy. If we cannot establish the right reasons for the patient's difficulties, after all, how can we be sure that a treatment programme is the right one for him? Often, unfortunately, it is not possible to be sure, and treatment has to proceed to a great extent in the dark. A wide range of treatment methods and programmes are available, and all have their successes and their failures. Some methods focus on the feedback problem (using delayed auditory feedback, cf. p. 58, or taking the patient's attention away from his speech by masking it (i.e. playing specially-generated 'noise' into his ears), cf. p. 120). Others focus on altering the patient's control of his breathing, or develop techniques in which he learns to speak more slowly and evenly than normal. Learning to relax is an essential feature of most methods, and several techniques are available to promote this. Learning to interact with others, especially in the situations which cause particular difficulty, is another essential feature of any remedial programme. If the stutter cannot be 'cured', it is argued, at the very least it can be brought more under the person's control, and the anxiety alleviated.

But in all these methods, the need for scientific study is pressing. As always, in clinical work, it is not the successes which need explaining, but the failures. Why did a certain treatment programme *not* succeed with an individual patient? To answer this question, accurate description of the formal characteristics of stuttering and of the contexts of its use is a necessity. Which sounds are more likely to be stuttered? in which parts of the word? in which parts of the sentence? during what kinds of speech activity? in spontaneous speech? in reading aloud? in reading the same passage aloud a second time? in talking to what kinds of people? to friends? acquaintances? strangers? superiors? in what kinds of situations? in shopping? on the telephone? The questions could fill up this page. The answers constitute a profile of the stutterer. Only by having many such profiles, spread over the natural history of the stuttering behaviour in many people, will the theoretical questions posed earlier in this section be resolved.[35]

But while the bulk of this section has to do with stuttering, it would be wrong to conclude that disorders of fluency are solely a function of that disorder. A further major category of nonfluency exists, known as *cluttering*. The primary characteristic here is the rapidity of the utterance: the patient attempts to talk too quickly, and as a result he introduces distortions into his rhythm and articulation. Sounds become displaced, misarticulated or omitted; words and partial words get repeated; syllables telescope into each other; the utterance comes out in relatively short bursts, often interfering with syntax; the speed may increase as utterance proceeds (a phenomenon known as *festination*). The description and theoretical study of cluttering is however less advanced even than that of stuttering. Once again, there is the need to take into account organic, personality, situational and other variables. The overlap between the categories of stuttering and cluttering should also be borne in mind: some patients present a mixture of both behaviours. It is possible that brain damage accounts for a greater proportion of clutterers (often, EEG recordings show significant abnormalities), but the evidence is by no means conclusive.

Lastly, it should not be forgotten that other types of speech pathology evidence abnormal fluency as part of the behaviour. Dysarthria, dyspraxia and dysphasia will all illustrate nonfluencies, ranging from mild to severe, and the same characteristics that we have discussed with reference to stuttering will be manifested—but this time as a secondary or derivative symptom.[36]

Voice disorders
The concept of 'voice', in popular usage, is a fairly general one, carrying a wide range of associations, such as when we interpret the variations in our

[35] See further, Dalton and Hardcastle, *op. cit.* and also C. W. Starkweather, *Fluency and stuttering* (Englewood Cliffs, Prentice-Hall 1987), L. Rustin, H. Purser & D. Rowley (eds), *Progress in the treatment of fluency disorders* (London, Taylor & Francis 1987).

[36] On cluttering, see D. A. Weiss, *Cluttering* (Englewood Cliffs, Prentice-Hall 1964), and Dalton and Hardcastle, *op. cit.*, Ch. 7.

voices as conveying emotions ('angry voice', 'sarcastic voice' etc.) or projecting our personalities ('young voice', 'depressed voice' etc.). Often the notion of voice relates to its aesthetic properties, and to someone's desire to improve their speech habits, by taking lessons in voice training (elocution). In speech pathology, however, a much more restricted sense is involved. Voice, and its associated disorders, refers to one of two variables, which have been labelled *phonation* and *resonance* (cf. p. 98). Phonation refers to the source of sound vibration in the vocal tract—primarily, therefore, the larynx. Resonance refers to the gross modifications of this vibration in the cavities contiguous to the larynx (i.e. excluding the fine modifications involved in articulation: see p. 99). Disorders of phonation therefore arise when something interferes with the normal functioning of the larynx, so that instead of the expected range of vocal effects (in pitch, voicing of consonants and vowels, and so on) noticeable distortions occur (such as hoarseness, or excessive breathiness). Disorders of resonance arise when something interferes with the functioning of the adjoining cavities (both beneath the glottis and above) so that abnormal timbres are introduced into the voice quality as a whole (as in excessively nasal voice).

There are many ways in which voice disorders can be classified, depending on whether we use medical, developmental, auditory or other criteria. One classification might look at the various growths which can appear on the vocal cords, for example, and treat them all together because, from a laryngological point of view, they form a single functional group. Another system might assign the lesions to different categories, depending on their etiology—for instance, lesions due to trauma (as in excessive use of the cords), those due to inflammatory causes (as with the result of laryngitis), and those of neoplastic origin (cf. p. 107). Another system might make a classification in terms of when the different growths were likely to appear (e.g. at puberty, in old age). Yet another might base itself on auditory criteria, grouping the lesions in terms of the kind of disturbance produced in the speaking voice (e.g. distinguishing different kinds of hoarseness). Each classificatory system has insights to offer the language pathologist, and aspects of each will be referred to below.

The language pathologist will naturally be interested primarily in the implications of the abnormality (whether organic or psychological—cf. below) for the way speech is affected. Not all lesions of the vocal tract, and certainly not all psychological states, affect voice quality: the language pathologist is only interested in those that do, or will. What are the main auditory effects likely to be produced by these lesions or states, therefore? Based upon our phonetic understanding of the variables involved (cf. p. 106), these effects can be grouped into three main types: abnormalities of pitch, of loudness, and of timbre. Under the heading of *pitch* would be included voices which were excessively high or low in pitch range, or involved excessively widened or narrowed range (with the maximum narrowing being reached with so-called 'monotone' voices). The vibratory level of pitch might also be affected producing, for instance, tremulous or over-vibrant qualities. There may also be an abnormal use of a pitch register (e.g. talking persistently in falsetto or excessively deep voices).[37] Under the heading of *loudness* would be included voices which were excessively loud or weak, or erratic in their control of loudness. Also included would be the effects of abnormally intense voice production on articulation—any general effects which characterized the whole of the patient's articulatory ability (such as a tendency for voicing to start too sharply at the beginnings of words, or to die away at the ends). Under the heading of *timbre* would be included the whole range of 'other' abnormal effects that affect the quality (as opposed to the pitch and loudness) of the tone (cf. p. 106). It is thus a very broad category, and it is usual to distinguish four types of vocal effect within it.

1 First, we must note the abnormal timbre that accompanies variations in the direction of the air-flow—if we speak while breathing in (cf. p. 95). Sometimes, noise is produced simply while breathing, with no attempt being made to speak; such noise is known as *stridor*, and is a feature of many laryngeal conditions.

2 Secondly, there is a range of specific phonation timbres produced at the larynx: the voice may emerge as a whisper, lacking any vocal-cord vibration; or vocal-cord vibration may be present, to some degree, but accompanied by excessive air-flow (a 'breathy' voice); or, there may be structural interference with the air-flow (e.g. due to the growth of abnormal tissue on the vocal cords) which will produce a 'hoarse' quality—a quality which will vary in its auditory effect, depending on the extent of the interference, and where in the vocal tract it takes place (e.g. whether parts of the lower pharynx are also affected). This group of timbre effects is collectively referred to under the heading of *dysphonia* or *aphonia* (the latter being used when there is no vocal-cord vibration present at all). Voices may be consistently or intermittently dysphonic or aphonic.

3 Thirdly, there is a range of abnormal resonance timbres, which may originate infraglottally (for instance, if the vital capacity of the lungs is reduced, as in lung or heart disease), or (more commonly) supraglottally: in this latter case, the main effects encountered are those which increase or decrease the amount of nasality present in the voice (an abnormally nasal, or 'twangy' voice (*hypernasality*); or a denasal voice (*hyponasality*)—common, for instance, in the sound of a blocked nose during a cold).

4 Fourthly, there are the abnormal timbres which result from alternative sources of phonation than the larynx. The most important ones to know about here are the result of the substitute voice-producing mechanisms which have to be learned as a result of laryngectomy (cf. p. 107). The

---

[37] It should be noted that we are here talking about the *phonetic* use of pitch, and not its phonological use, as in intonation. A patient may be speaking in an abnormally low pitch range, for example, but still making all the intonation contrasts of the language, e.g. distinguishing between questions and statements.

laryngectomee may be able to learn to use the upper part of his pharynx and esophagus to initiate vibration, and the resulting 'esophageal' and 'pharyngeal' voices are distinctive in their timbre. Alternatively, he may use an *artificial larynx* to provide him with a source of vibration—for instance a buzzing device which he places against the outside of his neck beneath his chin, while mouthing his speech. Again, a distinctive timbre is the result.

These are just the broad categories involved in the study of voice disorders. Each can be subclassified: for instance, several types of hoarseness and nasality have been proposed. The difficulty here, of course, is how to label them. Descriptive terminology for voice qualities is notorious for its ambiguity and vagueness. Take some of the terms for the description of hoarseness, for instance: 'wet', 'dry', 'rough', 'guttural', 'strident', 'metallic' and other such terms have been used in an attempt to characterize the auditory effects. At present, there is no consistent terminology, though several ongoing research projects are attempting to impose some order on the field.

A useful strategy to adopt when investigating the etiology of a voice condition is to ask three related questions: is the condition the result of abnormality in the normal course of physiological development? if not, is it the result of some organic damage to the vocal organs? if not, is it the result of psychological factors? In other words, we are here once again dealing with a process of diagnosis by exclusion. We can apply this reasoning to the above range of auditory variables.

Developmental disorders   There are several congenital disorders which will produce abnormal birth, hunger, etc. cries in the infant (abnormally formed vocal cords, for example (cf. p. 108), or disorders of chromosomal origin—a particularly dramatic example being the disorder known as *maladie du cri du chat*, 'cat-cry syndrome', so called because of the high whining sound the baby produces when it is crying).[38] At puberty, several abnormal things may happen to the voice during the period of adolescent change. In boys, instead of the normal process of *voice mutation* taking place, in which the voice becomes gradually lower, the prepubertal voice may stay, to produce an apparently falsetto effect known as *puberphonia*. In girls, the opposite effect may be found—an abnormally low or husky voice, which has been labelled *androphonia*. There could be a variety of causes for both disorders: the reasons may be organic (e.g. hormone imbalance, which in its extreme forms can result in gigantism, obesity, dwarfism, etc.) or psychological (e.g. a subconscious desire to 'sound' child-like, female, male etc., or a belief that the abnormal voice is pleasant, trendy, etc.—one recalls the low husky voices of several female film stars, for instance). And there are other possible causes—for instance, early cigarette smoking can produce an abnormally husky voice at this time in the female.

[38] The condition is the result of a partial or complete deletion of the short arms of chromosome number 5. Apart from the cry, infants are mentally retarded and display abnormal physical signs (such as abnormally small jaws or low-set ears).

Later developmental stages in adult life also can produce voice problems, particularly in the female, where menstrual function, climacteric (menopause) and pregnancy can all affect pitch, loudness and timbre, producing lower, weaker and harsher voice qualities in many women. Senescence is also a time when marked changes in voice characteristics occur, due to the normal degeneration of the vocal cords, and associated physiological and psychological changes. The laryngeal cartilages often stiffen, and the vocal cords become less elastic: reduced pitch range results, along with reduced loudness variation, tremulousness, variations in timbre and a generally reduced length of vocal performance.

Organic disorders   Voice disorders of organic origin can be related to the conventional medical categories referred to in Chapters 2 and 3. There may be structural abnormalities in the vocal tract, and affecting the vocal cords in particular. An important class is made up of *vocal nodules*, or *nodes*—a tiny bead of benign fibrous tissue on the margins of the vocal cords, usually bilateral and symmetrical, at the junction of the middle or anterior thirds of the cords. They are the result of excessive friction between the vocal cords— an irritative reaction to the mechanical trauma of over-using the voice. For this reason, they have been variously called 'singer's nodes', 'teacher's nodes' and 'screamer's nodes'. Medically, the condition is sometimes described as a localized 'chronic laryngitis', though the use of this term is felt to be inappropriate by some speech pathologists. If the nodes are allowed to develop, they become larger and firmer, and may result in the cords taking on an 'hourglass' appearance, because of the swellings on either side (see p. 108). The cords cannot therefore come together normally; their potential for vibration is thus affected; and the result is a marked hoarseness, tension and erratic voicing. The vocal strain which has produced this condition may be precipitated by various other factors, some physical (smoking, alcohol), some psychological (such as emotional stress). An interesting point is that the condition is about four times as likely to occur in women as in men, and is rare in children except between the ages of five and ten. The usual therapy is voice rest, perhaps for an extended period of time. Surgical removal of the nodes is also possible, but unless the cause of their appearance is eliminated, new nodes will re-emerge in due course. The patient will have to learn new techniques of managing his voice, if he hopes to prevent recurrence.

The other types of growth which may appear in the larynx also have their auditory consequences. Severe hoarseness may result from the development of papillomata (cf. p. 107), especially encountered in children in the first five years of life, and rare after the 30s. Polyps can produce a similar range of auditory abnormalities to nodules. Chronic hoarseness may be an early sign of carcinoma of the glottis, and is an important presenting symptom, as it can lead to early radiotherapy (which may remove the need for subsequent surgery). Contact ulcers may form as a result of the over-forceful adduction of the vocal cords, producing a very tense, low-pitched, hoarse or breathy voice, with an explosive quality. This condition, by contrast with vocal nodules, predominantly affects males, especially in middle age. As above, it is primarily due to misuse of the voice, but with the possibility of other factors having some influence (such as personality, or irritants, such as working in a smoky atmosphere, or smoking). As in all such cases, the therapist would want to check for the presence of these variables in the background of the patient.

Organic damage may result from several other factors: the direct trauma that results from injury to the larynx; the inflammations that may affect the larynx as a result of upper respiratory tract infections; the physiological disturbances in the endocrine system (in the thyroid and pituitary glands, for instance); the laryngeal signs of neurological damage, with the loss or weakening of vocal-cord movement on one or both sides (as in recurrent laryngeal nerve palsy and lower motor neurone disease, cf. p. 107). Each of these conditions produces a voice effect which combines abnormal pitch, loudness and timbre characteristics. With training, many of these conditions can be distinguished on the basis of their auditory signs, and changes in condition monitored by following the auditory changes as they occur. In such circumstances, the collaboration between speech pathologist and ENT surgeon is essential.

Psychological disorders   This concentration on developmental and organic voice disorders is to some extent an unreal emphasis. It has been estimated that over 70 per cent of the disorders which turn up in a voice clinic are due to causes other than these, i.e. psychological, or 'functional' (cf. p. 123). Three types of 'functional' etiology have been proposed. Firstly, there is the pattern of excessive use (*vocal abuse*), already described above, which can produce laryngitis, nodules, contact ulcers etc., and in which emotional and personality factors may be evident (a patient, for example, may have a long history of vocal abuse, but the development of lesions may be something which has taken place only recently, because of some additional emotional stress which has affected him). Secondly, there is the pattern of immature personality development, briefly mentioned above—a puberphonia developing, for example, because of a complex set of emotional or psychiatric reasons. The third category of psychological voice disorders has not been previously referred to, however, and these are perhaps best described as psychopathological in the sense of Chapter 3 (p. 68). In such cases, there is the development of a voice condition which is just as abnormal, auditorily speaking, as the organic conditions described above: there may be a complete loss of voice, varying degrees of dysphonia, abnormal nasality, pitch, loudness and so on. The commonest is referred to as *conversion aphonia* (or 'hysterical'/'functional'/'psychogenic' aphonia), in which in its extreme form the patient is able to speak only in a barely audible whisper; the vocal cords are incompletely adducting (though the patient can often cough, laugh, or cry well, showing that it is *speech* that is being primarily affected, and that there is no general paralysis of the larynx); the larynx is held rigidly, and speaking is abrupt, spasmodic; the voice is at times weak, at times harsh. The reason for the label was referred to in our discussion of psychoneuroses in Chapter 3: what seems to be happening is that the patient has lost control over her[39] (healthy) musculature because of an underlying emotional stress; her voice is symbolic of this stress (often a personal conflict in which communication difficulties between the patient and others have played a prominent part). It is argued that the patient is using her voice complaint as a means of not facing up to her emotional problems directly, and will usually deny that she has these problems, preferring to focus on the possibility that there is an organic cause for the complaint. Therapists repeatedly report a dramatic change in the patient's voice abilities, once she becomes able to recognize the underlying emotional cause; the patient may become quite emotional, once the therapist achieves a degree of rapport, and can persuade her to talk about her problems and to relax. The results may be quite rapid. Really deep-rooted psychoneurotic difficulties will however be beyond the skills of the speech therapist, and referral to a psychiatrist will be needed.

Other psychological dysphonias are recognized, and not all are fully understood. The importance of the therapist taking a full case history in such cases is crucial, if an accurate diagnosis is to be made, and appropriate management introduced. Information needs to be obtained under many headings: how long has the patient had the voice problem? has it been continuous or intermittent? have there been other voice problems? have there been voice problems in the family? have there been any recurring illnesses (especially affecting the respiratory tract)? where does the patient work? what are work surroundings like? are conditions noisy? how much does the patient use his voice? does he use the telephone much? does he smoke? drink? expose himself to other irritants? take drugs? These are but some of the headings that need to be gone through, before a complete picture can emerge. It is a procedure which is time-consuming and requires all of the therapist's professional and academic skills.

There is one other problem worth mentioning, as it has been implicit in everything that has been said in this section: voice disorders are, by definition, the abnormal aspects of the voice—but what, then, is a normal use of the voice? It may be intuitively easy to recognize a normal voice, i.e. one with no features which makes it stand out as unpleasant or interfering with communication; but what are the characteristics of the voice which make it normal? Surprisingly, this is a very difficult question to answer (cf. p. 9). We can say that a voice is normal if it is audible, clear, appropriate for the circumstances in which it is used (such as our job), gives the listener no sense of strain, and so on. But these are difficult notions to pin down. Who is to say if a voice is appropriate for a particular situation? Will

[39] It is primarily a female complaint, in the ratio of 7:1.

everyone agree about what makes for the 'best' voice, in a sermon, a public speech or a cocktail party? And above all, will the patient always agree with the therapist as to what constitutes a good, desirable voice? Most of us are quite happy to work on the assumption that we 'know' what a normal voice is, and there is usually sufficient agreement amongst clinicians to make the above question a rather academic one. But the uncertainty remains, and needs to be researched, and there are now some promising signs in the fields of social psychology and sociolinguistics that progress in defining the criteria of normality in voice use can be made.[40]

Disorders of articulation

This is the traditional centre of the speech pathologist's inquiry, involving the phonetic and phonological description and analysis of the patient's pronunciation. The notion of an articulation disorder is, however, a very wide-ranging one: at one extreme, it can refer to a completely misarticulated sound system, so that the person is largely unintelligible; at the other extreme, it can refer to a difficulty in a single sound or group of sounds (as with 'lisping', or 'weak' *r*). Classification of these problems is made, in the first instance, in terms of the normal parameters of phonetic description (cf. p. 103). From an anatomical (or 'structural') point of view, abnormal articulations can be identified at each of the possible 'places of articulation':

at the *lips*, e.g. the result of cleft lip (cf. p. 187), paralysis, or scar tissue;
at the *teeth*, e.g. the result of absent or misaligned teeth, or a deformity of the alveolar ridge;
at the *hard palate*, especially if cleft palate is involved;
at the *velum*, especially if poor contact is made with the pharyngeal wall;
using the *tongue*, e.g. the result of abnormality in its size or shape (after surgery, for instance, including the possibility of its total removal—the operation known as *glossectomy*);
in the *pharynx* and *larynx*, insofar as the articulation of sounds is concerned (as opposed to the phonation and resonance of voice, cf. p. 174).

It is not so much an abnormal anatomical structure which is the cause of misarticulation, however; indeed, it is often possible for the human vocal apparatus to compensate greatly for absent or malformed structures, and produce speech that is difficult to distinguish from normal speech. A more important factor is physiological incoordination, which can produce a general oral inaccuracy in sound production that may or may not be capable of being traced to neurological causes in encoding (dyspraxia, cf. p. 153) or

[40] This angle is well illustrated in H. Giles and R. St. Clair (eds), *Language and social psychology* (Oxford, Blackwell 1979). For a general introduction to the field of voice, the classical reference is M. C. L. Greene, *The voice and its disorders* (London, Pitman Medical, 4th edn. 1980). See also T. Bull and J. Cook, *Speech therapy and ENT surgery* (Oxford, Blackwell 1976); G. P. Moore, *Organic voice disorders* (Englewood Cliffs, NJ, Prentice-Hall 1971) and A. Murphy, *Functional voice disorders* (Englewood Cliffs, NJ, Prentice-Hall 1964); M. Fawcus (ed.), *Voice disorders and their management* (London, Croom Helm 1986).

transmission (dysarthria, cf. p. 155). Physiological factors are more pervasive because so many articulatory variables are involved: to get a sound right, the active articulator must be moved *in the right direction* towards the passive articulator, *at the right speed*, maintaining the *right shape*, making the *right amount of surface contact*, and maintaining the *right pressure*. If any of these variables are uncontrolled, the result will be a misarticulation, e.g. a fricative 'overshoots' and becomes a plosive; a plosive is delayed in its release phase and becomes an affricate; there is inadequate pressure to maintain an articulation, and the sound becomes erratic or weak. A particularly common cause is when one articulator fails to get released before the next articulation begins, as a result of which the auditory effect of the first articulation carries on through the rest of the syllable or word—as when the soft palate does not raise itself sufficiently quickly and the remaining articulations all become nasalized. Hearing loss is another factor which can disturb the ability to coordinate, discriminate and produce sounds.

We have already seen the amount of phonetic detail in which it is possible to specify the articulatory and acoustic identity of a sound. A great deal of articulatory skill is involved in producing, say, a [d] sound: the right part of the tongue (the blade) must be placed against the alveolar ridge (further back will produce auditory confusion, e.g. with [g]), along its whole horizontal extent (otherwise air would be released during the articulation and a hissy or breathy articulation would result); it must be placed there with a fair amount of muscular tension, in order to allow pressure of air to build up behind it in preparation for its release as a plosive sound (inadequacy here will produce a weak, indistinct articulation); the soft palate must be kept raised throughout the articulation (otherwise nasality will interfere, and the [d] will become [n]-like): there must be accurately-timed vocal-cord vibration—not too little (otherwise the sound will emerge as more [t]-like), and not too much (otherwise it will be 'over-voiced', emerging as a 'duh'). It should be plain from this brief description that there are several possible ways in which a [d] sound can 'go wrong'—and these are only some of the possibilities (I have not referred to the effects of simultaneously-occurring articulations elsewhere in the vocal tract). There are also several variations in the 'preferred' articulation of [d] in a given dialect, and this will need to be considered before an articulation can be considered as abnormal.

But in all this, an important point emerges: the approach as so far described is concerned to get the [d] sound *phonetically* correct; it is not directly concerned with the *phonological* status of the sound. In recent years, far more attention has come to be paid to the phonological implications of articulation problems. The change in emphasis can be summarized in this way. A phonological distinction, as we have seen (p. 41), is one where two sounds (or groups of phonetically similar sounds) have the role of distinguishing meanings in a language—for example, /p/ v. /b/ v. /d/ v. /s/ etc., as in *pin, bin, din, sin*. These are the phonemes of the language. Let us

take one of these—say /d/. There is in fact no single phonetic articulation of
this phoneme in normal speech: how /d/ is actually pronounced depends on
what sort of word it appears in, and where in the word it appears—a /d/ at
the beginning of a word is phonetically somewhat different from a /d/ at the
end of a word (it is more voiced in initial position, for example). These
phonetic differences do not affect the status of the phoneme: the sounds are
all recognized as variants of /d/—and would continue to be so recognized,
even if they were somehow mixed up (if you gave full voicing to /d/ in final
position, for instance, it would still be recognized as a /d/, though as a very
carefully articulated and emphasized one). Now, this principle carries
through into articulation disorders. There are many distortions which can
be given to the /d/ phoneme, as we have seen, but as long as they remain
within certain limits, they will be perceived as just that—/d/-distortions. If
they go over certain limits, however, then a different problem arises: if loss of
voicing becomes too great, the /d/ will emerge as a voiceless [t], and will thus
be confused with the /t/ phoneme. /din/ will now sound like *tin*, and not just
like a distorted version of *din*. One phoneme is now being confused with
another; the meanings of words is being directly affected; and we have a
phonological problem on our hands.

A purely phonetic articulatory problem is common enough: variations in
the articulation of /r/, /l/ and above all /s/ are cases in point. These only
rarely raise phonological problems: a person plainly has a defective /s/, and
there is no likelihood of it being confused with some other consonant or
vowel phoneme. Such problems, moreover, may never reach the speech
therapy clinic, being left to sort themselves out as a child grows up. What is a
more common, and also a more serious problem is when there is a limitation
in the patient's ability to express all the contrasts in his language's
phonological system. Either his phonetic inadequacy is so great that it has
blurred the distinctions between the phonemes; or, there is something wrong
with his underlying ability to organize his speech phonemically, and
phonetic confusion is one of the results. Let us look at some examples.

A common phonological problem is where the patient has only one sound
that he can make in a certain part of the mouth, and as a result all the
phonological contrasts which normally occur in that region are conflated.
One patient, asked to say *shoe*, said [tu:]; asked to say *Sue*, he said [tu:];
asked to say *two*, he said [tu:]; and so on. He was unable to make any
contrasts in the area between alveolar ridge and palate. Another had a more
confused system, with one phoneme 'overlapping' another in several places:

car /ka:/ was pronounced [ta:]
tar /ta:/ was pronounced [pa:]
pa /pa:/ was pronounced correctly.

At least here, the patient has a regular substitution pattern: he is replacing
one voiceless plosive by another—as if he has simply a 'misaligned' system.
Here is a more mixed-up case:

operation until after the first year or so, it will become increasingly difficult to correct the faulty patterns of articulation which will by then have become well established; on the other hand, if he intervenes in the earliest months, he must be sure to allow for the natural growth in facial processes yet to take place, so that his surgical correction does not interfere with this. Most cleft-palate operations in Great Britain are in fact performed within the first year of life; the prognosis for speech is therefore very promising.

What is the nature of the speech problems which result from the cleft palate syndrome? Obviously, articulation will be affected—and in particular those articulations which are made involving the lips and palate. But the situation is rather more complicated than this. Most aspects of articulation turn out to be affected, to some degree—the reason being that it takes time to develop the correct patterns of air-flow and muscular coordination required for smooth connected speech. If you have been breathing through your nose and mouth simultaneously for several months, and then find yourself having to operate with separate oral and nasal functions, the change in behaviour will not take place rapidly. There will be erratic control of the soft palate, and nasalization will affect many consonants and vowels. By losing air through your nose which you need for oral consonant articulations, many sounds (plosives and fricatives in particular) will be pronounced sloppily. It will be particularly difficult to keep up sustained pressure in the mouth, such as is needed for fricatives. Tactile feedback from the mouth may take time to be established, and there may be mis-articulation—the tongue overshooting or undershooting its targets. The transitions between sounds will be badly affected. Connected speech in particular will be unclear (as compared with producing single words in isolation).

But not only articulation will be affected. The way the patient makes his contrasts between sounds will be affected too (i.e. his phonology). If the operation has been left until after the beginning of his period of phonological development (not performed within the first two years), an idiosyncratic set of contrasts may have become established. Instead of saying *pin* and *bin*, the patient might have learned to say [in] and [ʔin] (i.e. to use a glottal stop instead of the voiced plosive). 'Unlearning' such substitutions may be quite complicated, even after the time when the real plosive contrasts are quite within his articulatory capabilities.

Voice production will also be affected—indeed, this is often the most dominant characteristic of cleft-palate speech. The voice becomes nasal (the exact quality depending on the type of cleft), and can be rated on scales running from mild to severe. There may be associated phonation disturbances—a husky voice, or a weakly-intoned voice, due to the increased incidence of upper respiratory tract infections in these patients (the incidence of mouth breathing promotes infection). This raises an additional complication: the infection moves via the Eustachian tube into the middle ear, resulting in otitis media (cf. p. 118). The middle ear may also be poorly aerated, because of poor muscular control of the tube's opening by the tensor palatini muscle (cf. p. 101). As a result, hearing problems are common in this group of patients: about half the population of cleft-palate patients have a bilateral loss of between 30 and 70 dB (depending on the extent of the cleft). It should also not be forgotten how much at risk these children are, especially when they are infants. There is a persistent risk of suffocation or pneumonia (due to inhalation of fluids). They are also a poor anaesthetic risk—and we must remember in this connection that some 40 per cent of cleft palates occur in conditions of multiple handicap (associated heart disorders, for example). Lastly, there is a real but unexplainable language delay with many of these children—presumably because of the interference from some of the factors already described, and the repeated institutionalization and emotional trauma which accompanies the condition. The amount of speech heard by the cleft-palate infant may also be down on normal: if one is being fed for six or eight hours a day, in the first months of life (feeding problems are inevitably very great), there is relatively little chance to play, to listen or to practice one's babbling.

In this field, as in all the others described in this chapter, there is plenty of research to be done. Detailed studies need to be made of the correlation between different types of cleft and phonetic and phonological behaviour. The results of using different surgical techniques and prosthetic devices (inserted into the cleft as a temporary measure) need to be evaluated precisely. At present, the many studies which have been made of the intelligibility or acceptability of cleft-palate speech after surgical intervention (after 3 months, 6 months, and so on) and after therapy are reduced in value by an inherent vagueness in the descriptive categories used. Which aspects of speech are being evaluated? For this, we need precise phonetic and phonological descriptions. How exactly do we rate such a notion as intelligibility? For this, more sophisticated psycholinguistic procedures need to be devised. [48]

Epidemiological issues

I have referred frequently throughout this chapter to the need for precise descriptions of the behaviour involved in linguistic disabilities, and for careful analysis of these behaviours in relation to the medical conditions underlying them. Without such information, it is difficult to arrive at any conclusions about the extent to which a disorder occurs within a population, and thus the extent to which there is a clinical need that has to be met—for instance, by the provision of special facilities within the health service. The science which deals with the prevalence, distribution and control of disease in a population is known as *epidemiology*, and in recent years, considerable

[48] Standard references are M. E. Morley, *Cleft palate and speech* (London, Churchill Livingstone, 7th edn. 1970), M. Edwards & A. C. H. Watson (eds), *Advances in the management of cleft palate* (Edinburgh, Churchill Livingstone 1980).

progress has been made in our understanding of linguistic disorders, from the epidemiologist's point of view; but there are several basic problems.

The question, 'How many cases are there of such-and-such a disease in the country?' is deceptively difficult to answer. Everything depends on how you identify the disease in the first place. How many speech defects are there? If by 'speech defects' you mean everything from the slightest detectable error in articulation to the most obvious forms of developmental disturbance, then your figure will be relatively high; on the other hand, if you mean only disorders of articulation, the figure will be much lower; and if you mean only those disorders of articulation which are sufficiently severe to need therapy, the figure will be lower still. Reviewing the literature on the prevalence of speech disorders, the Quirk Report concluded that about 3 per cent of children in ordinary schools suffered from some kind of speech disorder, but only about 2 per cent were in need of speech therapy. Age is another variable: in the preschool child, the Quirk Report concluded that nearer 3 per cent of children might need the services of a speech therapist (about 60,000 altogether, in 1972). A similar percentage has been suggested for the United States. An identical problem would face anyone interested in studying the prevalence of hearing loss in the community: how much hearing loss is included under this heading? under what kinds of circumstances? $2\frac{1}{2}$ per cent of the population is one estimate which has been given.

Such gross figures can be accumulated for any disease, if the information is available. There are many ways of obtaining the data—using interviews, analysis of case records, direct examination of samples, study of death registration records, and so on. In linguistic disorders, a factor which is of considerable importance is the adequacy of the medical history and the accuracy of the behavioural description. In so many cases, accurate accounts of medical and behavioural factors are lacking. This is one reason, it is said, why estimates of so many syndromes vary so much. Because birth records are often not clear, estimates of the cleft palate condition have ranged from 0·80 per 1000 to 1·70 per 1000 births. We can average this out and say that cleft palates are a little over one in 1000, and this is the figure usually quoted; but there is plainly a need for caution in interpreting this.

Such gross figures, also, are not necessarily the most interesting. Many people are more concerned, not with the overall statistics, but with a more detailed breakdown in terms of age, sex, social background, on the one hand, and type and degree of severity of the condition on the other. For example, it is important to know that in most speech disorders, boys are twice as likely to be affected than girls. In cleft palate, for instance, one study showed that for clefts of primary and secondary palate together, boys were more frequent than girls in a ratio of 2:1, whereas for clefts of the secondary palate only, the ratio was reversed. Unilateral primary clefts are more frequent than bilateral; clefts on the left side are more frequent than those on the right; clefts of the lip alone are likely to be less severe than when they occur in association with the palate; and there are several other such findings which can be of value to the clinician. For instance, it can give him some indication of the amount of treatment time which will need to be spent on follow-up work in a given area. Or it may give him a more realistic sense of the way research should be carried out. In one research study, into stroke patients, carried out at Northwick Park Hospital in Middlesex in the mid-1970s, 396 patients were admitted over a 2 year period. Of these, 31 per cent died; 16 per cent recovered quickly; and of the remainder, several had other illnesses, were too frail to be involved in a project, or simply lived too far away. The result was that only 51 (13%) of the patients that the project had hoped to study were able to be used. Being aware of such factors is an important prerequisite for planning and carrying out viable research.

Another important factor, in discussing these issues, is to ensure that a careful distinction is drawn between the notions of *prevalence* (which we have been discussing above) and *incidence*. Prevalence refers to the number of cases of a disease in a population at any given time. Incidence refers to the number of *new* cases of disease within a specific period (the 'attack rate'). This distinction is not just a terminological one: quite different pictures of a disease are obtained. For example, the incidence of acute otitis media (cf. p. 118) is 100 per 1000 of population per annum. However, the average duration of a case is only about a week, so that at any given time only 2 people in 1000 will be suffering from the disease.

The Quirk Report's (1972) estimates of the numbers needing speech therapy provides an interesting perspective for this chapter. No adult survey has taken place, so its figures are very much estimates:

	Total	% requiring speech therapy	Nos. requiring speech therapy
Geriatric patients	40,000	9	3600
Hospitalized stroke patients	16,000	?33	5000
Others (i.e. head injuries, voice disorders, stammerers, neurological cases etc.)	?30,000	100	30,000
		approaching	40,000

Estimates for children are more precise (England, Wales and Scotland only):

	Total		
Children in ordinary school	9 millions	2	180,000
ESN(M)	60,000	20	12,000
ESN(S)	35,000	50	17,500
Physically handicapped	12,000	25	3000
			212,500
Preschool	2 millions	3	60,000
			272,500

Other categories, such as partially-hearing children (cf. p. 130), autistic children etc. would increase this total still further. The Quirk Report concludes, as an 'informed guess' that well over 300,000 children and adults are in need of speech therapy services in this country—a figure which, it says, 'can err only in being too low' (78).

The contributing professions

Throughout this book, I have concentrated on presenting language pathology as an intellectual field of inquiry, which takes the data of clinical situations and attempts to provide a coherent frame of reference which will account for that data. Only on the basis of this, I have argued, is it possible to devise adequate procedures for screening, assessment, remediation, management and rehabilitation of the patient. A strong theoretical foundation is at all times essential, to guarantee consistency in the tasks facing the clinician (such as the description and analysis of patient behaviour) and to enable him to make headway in explaining awkward cases. It is not only the successful cases which a theory is called upon to explain, but also the failures: why has a remedial procedure *not* worked, in a specific instance? One of the themes of chapter 4 has been the distance which still has to be covered before any such comprehensive theory of linguistic pathology will be arrived at. The need to be critical of terminology, the search for analytic criteria, the concern for adequate data bases—these are issues which turn up repeatedly, as we move from the discussion of one disability to the next. Probably the biggest problem facing the language pathologist, though, is his need to integrate and interpret the findings from a multiplicity of different disciplines and academic traditions, each of which has an important contribution to make concerning linguistic disability. We have encountered several of these disciplines in the course of this book, as we reviewed the implications of working in medical and behavioural terms. It remains now to bring these disciplines together, in order to see clearly the academic breadth of the subject, and to anticipate what is involved when people talk about the 'team approach' to the investigation of linguistic disorders.

For those readers who are anticipating linguistic pathology as part of a career (in speech therapy, in particular), this perspective is very necessary. A common inquiry relates to the best kind of preliminary training needed in order to become an efficient speech clinician. It should be plain from the range of topics reviewed in this book, that there can be no single simple answer. Apart from the personal qualities necessary for successful clinical practice (a discussion of which falls outside the purview of this book), there are several academic and academically-inspired skills involved, which cut across the traditional division between arts and sciences. The two main foundation areas were reviewed in Chapter 2: medicine and the behavioural sciences. The former subject can be broken down into its main subdisciplines, of which the following would form the core of medical training in the various degree and diploma courses in the subject:

anatomy
physiology
neurology and neuropathology
oto-rhino-laryngology
pediatrics

orthodontics
plastic surgery
psychiatry
audiology

with some reference to embryology, genetics, general pathology and geriatrics. The behavioural sciences relevant to training are primarily linguistics and psychology. Under the heading of linguistics, we would expect to encounter courses in the following subjects:

phonetics and phonology
grammar
semantics
psycholinguistics (including language acquisition)
sociolinguistics

Under the heading of psychology, the following range of subjects would be relevant (though labels vary greatly, when one compares different courses):

developmental psychology
social psychology
cognitive psychology
perception
learning
individual differences

abnormal psychology
physiological psychology
methodology
applied psychology

Several other fields of study would make their appearance, including:

acoustics
educational theory
contemporary institutions (such as the health service, relevant aspects of the law, social services)
reading and writing skills
clinical administration and general practice
special modes of intervention (art, music therapy, etc.)

A range of other professionals would be involved from time to time, to put flesh on the concept of the team approach. These would include those people with whom the language pathologist must work, if he is to piece together a complete picture of the patient, such as:

educational psychologists
clinical psychologists
medical social workers
health visitors
school medical officers
general practitioners
physiotherapists

occupational therapists
orthoptists
teachers and remedial teachers
the child guidance service

All of these components would enter into the basic training of the clinician specializing in language pathology. None of them, though, it will be noticed, constitute the field of language pathology as such. Rather, they act as the contributory subjects on a synthesis of which the understanding and treatment of linguistic disability is founded. In each subject, apart from the learning of what is involved, separate attention must be paid to the *application* of its theoretical, methodological and empirical findings to the range of linguistic disorders that exist. Thus, alongside linguistics, in its various branches, there is the clinical application of these ideas to the various pathological areas—such as the use of grammatical or phonological models in carrying out assessments, or motivating remedial programmes. Alongside psychology, there are the various applications of that subject in relation to such problems as the evaluation of abnormal perception, social skills and emotional behaviour. And lastly, there is the coverage of the whole range of linguistic disabilities themselves, in which the contributory disciplines all play their parts: courses on aphasia, dysarthria, dyspraxia, and so on and so forth.

Faced with this enormous spread of subjects, it is essential to impose a conceptual order. No two courses are identical in their distribution of hours for the various components, nor in the themes which they single out for special attention. This is how it should be. One course may choose to devote extra time to clinical linguistic studies, another to applied psychological studies, another to educational applications, and so on. In a community where there is a strong bilingual element in the population, a course might well focus on the social and other problems which might promote linguistic disability and its remediation. But underlying all of these different emphases there is a unifying theme. It is well summarized in the Quirk Report (p. 72):

> . . . the would-be practitioner of therapy, whether of speech or hearing, of reading or of writing must in future regard *language* as the central core of his basic discipline. This does not, of course, imply that he may not opt for one rather than another speciality of interest among the various kinds of pathological manifestations. But the development of his particular skills ought to be along the lines of movement outward from the central core rather than occasional ad hoc excursions inward when problems of more than peripheral import occur.

It is in the spirit of this recommendation that this book has been written.

5

Current trends in language pathology

In the decade which has elapsed since the first edition of this book, there has been a remarkable increase in the number and range of publications within the field of language pathology—a development which is reflected in the increased extent of the bibliography on p. 215. All levels of exposition have been affected, from basic popularization to research monograph, and several new specialized journals—always a sign of major growth in a subject—have appeared, such as *Clinical Linguistics & Phonetics*, *Aphasiology*, and *Child Language Teaching and Therapy*. At the same time, the phenomenon of language disability has received a more distinctive image, following persistent publicity from national charities and professional bodies about the range of conditions involved, and fresh survey data about the extent of language disability in the population and the numbers of professionals available to deal with it. Concern over matters of professional status and pay has also been a dominant theme of the 1980s, and this has played its part in focussing public attention on the existence of the problem of language handicap and its treatment. On the other hand, there is long way to go. In a survey of the general public carried out in 1987 by a US public relations firm on behalf of the American Speech-Language-Hearing Association, it emerged that fewer than one in five people knew exactly what a speech therapist did, and fewer that one in ten were familiar with the work of an audiologist.[1]

During the 1980s, the most important developments in the study of language disability took place within the range of disciplines categorized on p. 27 as 'behavioural'. This is not of course to diminish the importance of innovative medical techniques which came to be used in this field during the period. Aphasiology, for example, saw the implementation of new kinds of brain scan using nuclear magnetic resonance (NMR), which is a major step forward in the techniques referred to on p. 88; and the

[1] Burson-Marsteller Public Information Survey, *Asha* 29 (8), 1987, 21-5. For other statistical information about incidence and provision in Britain, see A. Webster, 'The prevalence of speech and language difficulties in childhood', *Child Language Teaching and Therapy* 4 (2), 1988; P. Enderby & R. Philipp, 'Speech and language handicap: towards knowing the size of the problem', *British Journal of Disorders of Communication* 21 (2), 1986, 151-65.

field of deafness saw great progress in the use of cochlear implanting (cf. p. 119). But these individual developments are of a different order from the fundamental way in which our perceptions of language disability have been altered by the application of ideas from the fields of psychology and linguistics. It is too soon to be certain, but there are signs that the progress in this domain made during the 1980s may prove to be comparable to that which came from the development of the medical model by neurologists in the late 19th century.

The thrust of much of the early work within the behavioural model was to provide exact descriptions of the linguistic symptoms presented by people suffering from the range of clinical conditions outlined in Chapter 4—comparable in their precision and comprehensiveness to the descriptions of disease which have long been available using the medical model. Each of the main dimensions of the view of language presented on pp. 40-47 was systematically investigated during the late 1970s and early 1980s, in a sequence which broadly corresponded to the way in which these dimensions had been studied in normal language acquisition in children a decade previously. Phonological analyses were among the first to be made, plotting the abnormal patterns of vowels, consonants, and syllables found in different types of patient, and suggesting factors which might account for the kinds of variation observed. At the same time, grammatical analyses were made of abnormal sentence constructions and word formations, many of which were related to the developmental patterns found in child language studies (during this period, also an area of unprecedented growth). The many aspects of semantic analysis also progressed, notably with reference to patterns of limited or unbalanced vocabulary growth, and to difficulties in producing or comprehending the underlying patterns of meaning in sentences and sentence sequences. One area where there was relatively little progress was in the study of the abnormal use of intonation, rhythm, tone of voice, and other aspects of *nonsegmental* phonetics and phonology (p. 41)—a domain which is traditionally a neglected branch of language study. An important exception was the analysis of the phonetic properties of voice quality, where the first successful attempts were made to replace the vague impressionistic terminology of voice disorders (p. 175) with a more objective, exact, and systematic description.[2]

---

[2] The various branches of this field are reviewed in D. Crystal, *Clinical linguistics* (London, Edward Arnold, 1987), C. Code and M. Ball (eds.), *Experimental clinical phonetics* (London, Croom Helm, 1984), and in Vol. 1 (1) of *Clinical Linguistics & Phonetics* (Basingstoke, Taylor & Francis, 1987). The background to the voice quality research is given in J. Laver, *The phonetic description of voice quality* (Cambridge, CUP, 1980), and an account of the clinical voice profile in the University of Edinburgh Department of Linguistics Working Papers, Vol. 14 (1981).

Pragmatics

An unmentioned topic in the figure on p. 46 came to prominence in the late 1980s—the domain of *pragmatics*. Conceptually, one may locate this topic in an area 'between' language structure and language use:

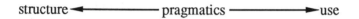

structure ◄————— pragmatics ————————►use

Pragmatics is the study of the factors which govern our *choice* of language (the sounds, constructions, words) in social interaction, and the effects of our choice upon others. The subject includes the analysis of what it means to be appropriate and cooperative in our speaking behaviour, and it thus begins to explain what is involved when we use language to convey politeness, intimacy, playfulness, rudeness, awkwardness, and a range of other 'social' attitudes. It is a truism that many patients have difficulty in using language appropriately; what is less obvious is why this happens. Typically, children who have a good command of language but a poor command of language use are given a wide range of impressionistic and often misleading descriptions: I have heard them called 'confused', 'awkward', and 'obstinate'; one was described critically with the words, 'he's always trying to be funny'; another with 'he just won't cooperate'. Now while there are undoubtedly many children for whom these words would be an apt description, there are also many for whom they miss the point entirely. It is so easy to assume that those who use language inappropriately are displaying a perverse attitude, especially if they have an excellent command of language structure. But it is gradually becoming apparent that there are many children whose behaviour is not under conscious control, and who are genuinely handicapped by an inability to understand and control the way in which language is used in everyday interaction. These are the children who have been referred to as having a 'pragmatic disorder', or, when seen in the context of an accompanying difficulty of vocabulary and comprehension, a 'semantic-pragmatic disorder'. A similar functional inadequacy can also be seen in some adult patients, notably in the more 'fluent' kinds of aphasia and in certain psychopathological conditions (such as schizophrenia).

It is important to appreciate that these children display a wide range of symptoms, and that at present it is not possible to generalise about the condition. There are many anecdotes about how the children behave, but few detailed case studies. Plainly there exists a continuum of pragmatic handicap, ranging from children who say little or nothing to those who talk normally. At one end of this continuum, there are those who are completely unwilling to engage in conversation, and who are totally unresponsive to the demands of normal social interaction. They may, to all extents and purposes, appear mute. Somewhat less extreme are children who are responsive, in a limited way, but not very assertive; they will talk when spoken to, but will not initiate a conversation themselves. Then, further along the continuum, there are those who are willing to engage in conversation, but who introduce their own rules, such as bringing in bizarre or irrelevant topics, answering their own questions, echoing what has just been said, not listening to what has just been said, talking too much, or changing the subject in unexpected ways. And lastly, at the near-normal end of the extreme, there are children who carry on a generally normal conversation, but who occasionally introduce a remark which is 'odd' (e.g. asking 'why?' at the wrong place), sounding rather stereotyped, or failing to cope when someone uses language in a special way (e.g. when people are 'kidding' or being sarcastic).

The following examples illustrate just a few pragmatically abnormal interactions. (It is important to emphasise that some of these examples could occur in normal children or adults—for example, when they are not paying attention, or are temporarily confused. A diagnosis of pragmatic disorder would be appropriate only when an accumulation of similar instances presented a general picture of inappropriate language use.) In the first, P does not answer the question, and keeps straying from the point:

T 'where do you 'go to schòol/
P Tòmmy 'goes to mý 'school/ because I 'see him in the 'hall everydày/ but we have 'different tèachers/ and 'he has a 'new bìcycle/

In the next case P seems unable to see the point of T's question:

T thàt's a 'nice pícture/ — can you téll me a'bout it/
P yès/ *silence*
T well 'go ón then/ tèll me a'bout it/

In the next, P says something which he couldn't really know, as T hasn't told him what the games are yet:

T will you 'play some gámes 'with me/
P yês/
T they're 'very èasy gámes/
P they 'are indèed/

In the following case, P imitates T, inappropriately:

T (*greeting the headteacher*) good mòrning 'John/
P good mòrning 'John/

Here, P takes T literally:

T 'take this 'note to Mr Smìth's 'room/

   P   *obediently goes to Mr Smith's room and returns still carrying the note*

In the following sequence, things get really confused:

   T   which ràce would you 'like to be 'in/
   P   I 'like to be in Blànktown at the spórts day/
   T   in Blànktown/
   P   yès
   T   what do you mèan/
   P   I mèan sómething/
   T   'is there a spòrts day in 'Blankschool/
   P   there is nòt/
        there is a 'sports day in Dàshschool/
   T   then what's Blànktown 'got to 'do with it/
   P   nòthing/
   T   then whý did you mèntion it/
   P   in'deed I dìd 'mention it/
   T   whỳ did you 'mention it/
   P   I don't knòw/

And, as a last example, a further piece of inappropriateness:[3]

   P   *(meeting the author as he arrives at P's school)*
        helló/ are 'you 'Professor Crỳstal/
   A   yès/
   P   mỳ name is 'J— 'K—/ I have to 'take you to 'see the headmàster/
   A   thànk you/ 'which way ìs it/
   P   'down hère/ *(they begin to walk)*
        do you lìke being márried/

The interaction between levels

While it is possible to find patients whose ability to control linguistic structure is excellent and whose problems are solely pragmatic in character, it is far more usual for them to display a mixture of difficulties. Most patients who present with pragmatic symptoms have linguistic problems too, such as a poor command of the way verbs are used, or a difficulty in stringing sentences together in a narrative. The structural and pragmatic aspects of the handicap, one would now say, *interact* in various ways. This emphasis on the interaction between the different aspects of linguistic disability is something which came very much to the fore in the 1980s. The language model on p. 40ff., however, does not reflect this: rather, it shows the way clinical linguistics was developing in the 1970s, where a great deal of attention was devoted to a detailed analysis of

---

[3] Several of the above examples are taken from published studies; some are from my own files. See further, M. McTear, *Children's conversation* (Oxford, Blackwell, 1985, Chapter 9), T.M. Gallagher & C.A. Prutting (eds.), *Pragmatic assessment and intervention issues in language* (San Diego, College-Hill Press, 1983).

individual levels of language. An account would be given of the patient's phonological ability, with no reference being made to other (grammatical, semantic, pragmatic) domains; or a patient's grammar would be studied independently of phonology and semantics; and so on.

In cases where it is plain that only one level is affected (as in a simple kind of articulation problem), this focus would not be misleading; but in the majority of cases, such simplicity does not obtain. The language of most children with developmental disorders or of most adult aphasics is a mixture of symptoms that can be located at different linguistic levels; and the question of how they interact thus immediately arises. We can elect to examine the grammatical aspect of the problem alone, or the phonological aspect, in just the same way as a doctor can investigate one part of the body while temporarily ignoring other parts; but before arriving at a linguistic diagnosis, the language clinician would be wise to bear the medical model in mind, with its proper emphasis on the ultimate need to consider the way the body functions in an integrated, balanced manner. In language, as in the body as a whole, what happens in one domain may affect the functioning of another domain. The linguistic evidence is slowly accumulating, both in normal child language studies and in clinical studies, that a great deal of interaction between levels of language organisation is routine, and may be an important element in the diagnosis of language disability.

As an example, we may consider the following dialogue between a therapist and a child patient aged 4½, whose grammar was close to that of a 2-year-old. Therapy had been proceeding on building up a Subject-Verb (e.g. *the boy is eating*) and Verb-Object (*kick a ball*) sentences, and had been succeeding. The child's vocabulary was also limited, for his age, but he was known to have about 200 words, and the therapist decided to elicit a three-element sentence of Subject-Verb-Object (such as *the boy is kicking a ball*), and part of the dialogue went like this:

```
T    'what's the 'boy dòing/
P    'kicking a bàll/
T    that's rìght/ he's 'kicking a bàll/ the 'boy's 'kicking a bàll/ — whát's
     'happening/
P    'kicking a bàll/
T    whò is/
P    a bòy/
T    yês/ 'can you 'say the 'whole thíng/
P    'him kìcking/
T    whò's 'kicking/
P    the bòy/
T    'what's the 'boy dòing/
P    'kicking the bàll/ ... ...
```

This kind of conversation proceeded for some time, with P 'evading' the complete form of the sentence which T was trying to get him to say. Finally, he tried it, with the following result:

P   he — 'him 'boy ki — 'kicking a bàll/
T   góod bòy/ 'say it agáin/ whát's he 'doing/
P   [dum]'boy bi — 'bicking a a bàll/

What is of note here is the way P's pronunciation deteriorates as he tries for the more complex sentence: the word *kicking* is affected by the surrounding [b] sounds; a nonsense word comes in ([dum] may be a blend of *the* and *him*); and the child becomes really quite non-fluent. In some cases, attempting a complex sentence can cause a noticeable stutter— something which has often been heard in normal children as they pass through certain grammatical stages (p. 168). The dialogue thus illustrates the existence of an interaction between phonology and grammar, and incidentally indicates how careful a clinician has to be in pacing language training.

It is not yet clear what is happening when patients display effects of this kind, whether between phonology and grammar, phonology and semantics, grammar and semantics, or any other combination. There may be a general constraint which limits the amount of linguistic complexity it is possible for the brain to process at any moment; or perhaps some components of language are more central than others, or more easily disrupted. One of the most important current developments in psycholinguistics is the construction of models of brain function which interrelate the linguistic components in different ways. Using these models, it is then possible to suggest hypotheses about the form language should take when one component is impaired, and to test these hypotheses in experiments or by analysing language samples. Commonly, these models also incorporate the elements thought to be involved in the process of reading and writing.[4]

Clinical linguistic diagnosis

From this account, the proper explanation of a patient's linguistic symptoms is a complex and time-consuming process, in which a language sample has to be analysed into its various levels of organization, the interactions determined, and the rules governing the competence of the impaired speaker deduced. To engage in clinical linguistic diagnosis is a truly professional task, and to be successful it requires a degree of training, time, resources, status, and pay for its practitioners which one

[4] There is a review of the literature on the interaction between levels in D. Crystal, 'Towards a 'bucket' theory of language disability: taking account of interaction between linguistic levels', *Clinical linguistics & phonetics* 1(1), 1987, 7-22. For the psychological issues involved, see M. Harris & M. Coltheart, *Language processing in children and adults: an introduction* (London, Routledge & Kegan Paul, 1986), and A. Ellis, *Reading, writing and dyslexia: a cognitive analysis* (London, Erlbaum, 1984)

would associate with any complex area of enquiry. Unfortunately, as language clinicians and teachers know only too well, it is rare to find all these elements being satisfactorily recognised, and thus it is routine to encounter teaching and therapy taking place where it has been possible to engage in only a minimum of analysis. It is not surprising, then, to hear complaints from professionals that they do not have the time to practise the techniques associated with the behavioural model of investigation, apart from in a few special settings, such as residential speech and language schools or university speech therapy clinics.

The solution to this problem goes well beyond the brief of the present book, involving a wide range of political and professional issues. But it is important to stress that no solution will be found if it ignores the clinical realities of the nature of language disability. Given the demonstrable enormous complexity of human language, it should be no surprise to discover that language disabilities are also complex, and require correspondingly complex intervention procedures. The professions have already come to recognise the inadequacies in the traditional clinical picture. The 1980s saw a gradually increasing dissatisfaction with established clinical labels (such as *dyspraxia*, *delay*, *aphasia*), and a demand for more discriminating categories. This is of course what led in the first place to the emergence of the more sophisticated linguistic and psychological approaches referred to above, and associated developments in assessment and teaching procedures. The irony is that intellectual conviction does not guarantee routine implementation. Because it is often not possible, for practical reasons, to introduce these new approaches, many centres continue to use routinely the established labels, tests, and materials. There has thus emerged a considerable, undesirable gap between clinical theory and practice.

Moreover, there are signs that this gap is not yet at its widest. One of the most persistent demands of the 1980s was for measures to be devised which would demonstrate the *efficacy* of therapeutic intervention. The questions were often asked: 'What value is speech therapy or remedial language teaching?' 'Can it be proved that therapy works?' It *is* possible to provide satisfactory and positive answers to such questions, but only after a great deal of effort has been expended. As with the medical model, the task is simply (sic) to keep meticulous records of all the relevant variables while therapy is in progress. After all, if patient A has no use of a structure, X, which should have been acquired two years previously, and a therapist works on that structure in a specific way for a specific period of time, and A then begins to use X, one would be perverse not to attribute at least some of the credit to the therapy. But to *prove* that this is what happened, one would need to have a convincing description of A's language at the beginning of therapy (to show that structure X was absent), another description of A's language at the end (to show that it was present), and a further description of what went on in between (to show that the teaching was relevant). Many such 'longitudinal' case studies of clinical intervention are needed before it will be possible to draw general conclusions about the efficacy of therapeutic techniques, and to begin to think predictively about therapy (i.e. to answer the question 'How much and what kind of therapy does it take to instill a particular structure into a particular type of patient?'). Few such studies have been carried out, mainly because of the amount of effort involved in making the multiple descriptions and analyses of what are always several linguistic variables.

There is, moreover, a further dimension to the diagnostic task for language clinicians, namely, to ensure that the linguistic foundation that they may establish in a patient at a particular point in time stands up under the weight of the language demands made on that patient in later years. This is a factor which is in principle relevant for patients of any age, but it is of particular concern with young children, whose language must take them through the educational system. The problem can be highlighted using the case of a 5-year-old child with a history of language delay. He has been receiving speech therapy for some time, and this has enabled him to catch up sufficiently that he is now able to cope with the demands placed upon him during his first year at school. What is the prognosis? Will he be able to keep up by himself during the remainder of his primary school? Or will he need further therapy? Will his reading and writing be affected? Or his number work? Current theory does not give us the answer to such questions, so at the very least we would need to monitor that child's subsequent language development. But for how long? It can be seen straight away that a commitment to a substantial period of follow-up study is required if we are to be sure that the language problem has 'run its course', or, correspondingly, if we are to discover the areas of weakness which will emerge as the child attempts to learn the more advanced kinds of language which he will encounter while he is in junior and senior school. The time-scale of a language disability is an integral part of its definition (just as, in the medical model, the time it takes for a disease to run its course is an integral part of the disease), and we cannot arrive at a final diagnosis until we have some longitudinal information to take into account.

A full clinical linguistic inquiry is thus a major enterprise, involving the description and analysis of the patient's language at several points in time, and also of the kind of language being used to the patient by the various adults (and perhaps other children) who have a caring role. The complexity is no greater, in principle, than that which is encountered in medical diagnosis. In practice, however, the two domains are worlds apart. If behavioural studies of language disability had the range of resources corresponding to the hospital pathological laboratory and the medical hierarchy (from general practitioner to hospital consultant), the situation would be drastically different.[5]

[5] The argument of this section is developed at length in D. Crystal, *Linguistic encounters with language handicap* (Oxford, Blackwell, 1984).

The broader context

The above discussion has focussed fairly narrowly on the way in which the linguistic component of the behavioural model has come to be refined in the 1980s, under the general heading of *clinical linguistics*. At the same time, there has been a move away from a narrow linguistic focus, with language being seen in the broader context of the whole range of cognitive and social skills presented by the patient. In the wake of various government reports, primarily on the 'special needs' of children, the emphasis has come to be more on the 'whole patient', and the notion of the 'team' of specialists has come to the fore. This wider context presents many new issues for consideration. How does a team approach to language actually work in practice? How are people trained so that they become aware of the professional expertise of other members of the team? How far is it possible to be precise in making statements of need, when it comes to working with language?

Such questions have come to be repeatedly addressed in other works, and have provided a stimulating perspective for the fresh discussion of traditional issues in language disability and the nature of the handicap which stems from it. Moreover, this perspective has generated renewed interest in several topics which had traditionally been considered somewhat marginal. The first is the range of problems associated with the *bilingual* child with language disability. Although there is a widely held popular view to the contrary, there is no necessary language handicap associated with being bilingual; indeed, probably the majority of children in the world grow up in a multilingual environment, and it is easy to underestimate the number of children involved, even in a relatively monolingual society such as Britain, as over 100 foreign languages are used by substantial numbers of immigrant people. On the other hand, there is no denying that there are many situations where children can be disadvantaged by their bilingual situation, especially if this is associated with strong and conflicting ethnic sensibilities (as in the case of many immigrant families), and the problem can take on a clinical dimension, often psychological and social as much as linguistic.[6] In addition, one would expect to find within the bilingual population the usual range of language-handicapping conditions—the problem being that in such circumstances these will be especially difficult to identify and treat. The task thus requires the adoption of a very broad perspective, involving social, cultural, educational and other factors; and it is undoubtedly an area which is now attracting a great deal of attention, in which several speech therapists and remedial language teachers have chosen to work. At the same time, fresh research tasks present themselves, such as the need

[6] On clinical aspects of bilingualism, see N. Miller (ed.), *Bilingualism and language disability* (London, Croom Helm, 1984). For the bilingual situation generally, see S. Abudarham (ed.), *Bilingualism and the bilingual* (Windsor, NFER-Nelson, 1987) and E. Harding & P. Riley, *The bilingual family: a handbook for parents* (Cambridge, CUP, 1986).

to adapt techniques of assessment and intervention to the cultural milieu of the immigrant patient.[6]

My second example is in the field of alternative and augumentative communication. For a very large number of children and adults, the normal use of spoken language is out of the question, because of the gross nature of their physical or mental handicap. Signing and other forms of communication have long been in use (pp. 135-7), as have simple mechanical devices used for pointing at letters, words, or symbols on a chart. But in the 1980s there was a marked interest in the potential of several kinds of system using signs and symbols, and the technological progress which followed the electronic revolution of the 1970s altered the educational scene. In some countries, the effects can be seen on television every day, in the form of sub-titled programmes for the deaf. But this is only the tip of a vast iceberg of innovation involving the new technology, which affects the lives of many speech-handicapped people, such as those suffering from cerebral palsy, aphasia, voice disorders (laryngectomees, in particular), and mental handicap.

The growth in the field of communication aids is one of the noticeable developments of the decade, and considerable effort has come to be devoted to assessing the residual abilities of a person so that the best choice can be made of a device which will enable them to achieve their maximum communicative potential. These devices include various types of voice output aids that can be programmed with a specific number of words and phrases or in which speech can be generated 'sound by sound' by typing in letters from a conventional keyboard. For those with learning difficulties, there are now several home- or school-based interactive computer-aided instruction systems, using video materials. And great progress has been made in the design of portable communication aids, based on visual or tactile systems of communication, in which messages are signalled by pointing to different parts of a chart or screen, using whatever part of the body over which there is some degree of motor control (which may be as limited as a head jerk or eyebrow movement). In all cases, the aim is to broaden the horizons of the handicapped person, to give a greater measure of independence and freedom, and increase educational opportunity. Often, these devices have been the means whereby a person's latent literary creativity can be expressed for the first time. 'Modern technology' wrote one such person, 'has allowed me to release my creative spirit where it can soar, free, high above the clouds. Without the fruits of modern technology, I would probably be stuck in a room counting the hours until my death'. It is easy for non-handicapped people to forget the way a speech-handicapped person's life can be fundamentally changed by having such equipment available. However, the success stories which receive most publicity should not be allowed to obscure the way in which practical factors (such as cost) interfere with the ideal. There are still very many adults and children whose communicative potential continues to be held back because they, or those who care for them, are unable to afford the equipment.

The electronic revolution has dramatically altered the lives of speech handicapped people, and will continue to do so, as more sophisticated forms of natural language processing become available. And this revolution is also likely to have dramatic effects on the lives of those who work with language disability, both in research and therapy. It is now possible to process complex data from devices which monitor speech movements, and to represent the activity on a visual display unit; an example is the technique for plotting tongue contacts against the palate, the *electropalatograph* (itself a development of 1980s' phonetics research). Several of the more complex language analysis procedures referred to earlier in this chapter are now available in computational form. The tiresome counting-up and comparison of items belonging to different language samples can now be much reduced by using various clinically-oriented software packages. And a wide range of teaching programmes is available on video, providing children with a highly motivating learning situation. It is not yet possible to pass all the labour of clinical language investigation onto the microprocessor: it will be some time before advances in automatic speech recognition, for example, will make it unnecessary for therapists to transcribe their tape samples. And many of the new software packages need to be used with caution, as they suffer from all the 'bugs' that one has come to associate with any new computational development. But the outlook is promising, and there are many who feel—this author among them—that the problems presented by the complexity of clinical language analysis will be considerably alleviated by appropriate, clinically sensitive computational techniques, in all areas of language pathology—diagnosis, assessment, screening, and remediation.[7]

[7] Several introductions to this field are now available: J.F. Curtis, *An introduction to microcomputers in speech, language and hearing* (Boston, College-Hill Press, 1987); D. Hawkridge, T. Vincent & G. Hales, *New information technology in the education of disabled children and adults* (London, Croom Helm, 1985), and A.H. Schwartz (ed.), *Handbook of computer applications in communication disorders* (San Diego, College-Hill Press, 1984). For the general background of ideas in computer science, see D. Rowley & H. Purser, *Clinical information technology* (London: Taylor & Francis, 1988). For reviews of specific programmes, see the Computer Applications section in each issue of *Child Language Teaching and Therapy*.

On the nature of alternative and augmentative communication, see R.L. Schiefelbusch (ed.), *Nonspeech, language, and communication: analysis and intervention* (Baltimore, University Park Press, 1980); C. Kiernan, B. Reid & L. Jones, *Signs and symbols: use of non-vocal communication systems* (London, Heinemann, 1982); and the various issues of *Augmentative and Alternative Communication* (Baltimore, Williams & Wilkins).

Appendix

Some common names and abbreviations

A wide range of psychological, pediatric and linguistic tests are available for the assessment of the handicapped child and adult. The following are some of those in common use, which the student of language pathology is likely to encounter early on in the observation of clinical and teaching situations.

Aphasia Screening Test (AST), by R. Whurr, is a battery of tests for use with adult aphasics; it consists of 20 receptive and 30 expressive tests, and provides a profile of eight language components: visual perception, reading comprehension, reading aloud, auditory comprehension, speech production, oral language, writing, and calculation.

Aston Index, by M. Newton and M. Thomson, is a classroom test for screening and diagnosis of language difficulties, for use with children between 5 and 14; it contains 6 tests of general ability, which result in a mental age score, and ten performance tests which examine skills specifically required for the acquisition of written language.

Auditory Discrimination Test (revised 1973), by J. W. Wepman, uses a series of word pairs designed to test whether children (between 5 and 8) can discriminate English phonemes.

Boston Diagnostic Aphasia Examination, by H. Goodglass and E. Kaplan, is a series of tests which assess the type and severity of adult aphasia using profiles of conversational and expository speech, and tests of auditory comprehension, oral expression, written comprehension, and writing.

British Ability Scales are a series of 24 tests which assess a wide range of cognitive abilities, such as reasoning, short-term memory, and perceptual matching; they are used with children between 2½ and 17, and have been standardized on a British population.

British Picture Vocabulary Scale, by L. M. Dunn, L. M. Dunn & C. Whetton, is a test of listening vocabulary, standardized on a population between 2½ and 18 years; published in 1982, it has largely superseded the earlier *English Picture Vocabulary Test*.

Clinical Language Intervention Programme (CLIP), by E. Semel and

E. H. Wiig, involves the assessment and training of a wide range of linguistic skills in semantics, syntax, memory, and pragmatics; for use with 5- to 13-year-olds.

Coloured Progressive Matrices, by J. C. Raven, is a series of tests designed to assess the intellectual abilities of people with linguistic, physical or mental handicaps; especially usable with children between 6 and 11 and with the aged.

Derbyshire Language Scheme, by M. Masidlover & W. Knowles, is a series of assessments of a child's expressive and receptive language, linked to a programme of teaching activities designed to develop linguistic abilities; it is aimed especially at children with a language age below 4½.

Distar is an abbreviation for 'Direct instruction system for teaching and remediation', a US series of lessons for use with children between 5 and 8, with components on language, reading, and arithmetic.

Draw-A-Man Test, by F. Goodenough, is an intelligence test based on a child's ability to draw a person, paying attention to accuracy and detail rather than creative ability.

Edinburgh Articulation Test (EAT), by A. Anthony, D. Bogle, T. T. S. Ingram and M. W. McIsaac, involves the articulation of 77 items in 41 words, assessed quantitatively and qualitatively, for use with children between 3 and 6 years.

English Picture Vocabulary Test (EPVT), by M. A. Brimer and L. M. Dunn, is a test of listening vocabulary; it contains a series of pictures, printed in groups of four, from which the child must select one in response to a verbal cue; used from age 3 to adulthood. See also *British Picture Vocabulary Test.*

Frenchay Aphasia Screening Test (FAST), by P. Enderby, V. Wood & D. Wade, is a quick screening test, designed at the Frenchay Hospital, Bristol, in which patients respond to a small range of pictures and sentences; it is designed to help non-specialists refer patients suspected of having aphasia to speech therapists.

Frenchay Dysarthria Assessment, by P. Enderby, is a procedure designed at the Frenchay Hospital, Bristol, which rates dysarthric speech in terms of a range of oral, facial, and speech tasks; it derives a profile of ability which can be used to discriminate types of dysarthric speakers, and provide a basis for management.

Frostig Developmental Test of Visual Perception tests the perceptual skills of young children in five areas: eye motor coordination, figure ground, consistency of shape, position in space, and spatial relationships; especially used for children with learning difficulties and neurological handicaps.

Functional Communication Profile (FCP), by M. Taylor-Sarno, assesses an adult aphasic's functional communicative abilities, using a list of 45 everyday contexts.

Goldman-Fristoe Test of Articulation is an American test, by R. Goldman and M. Fristoe, which assesses the articulation of consonants and consonant clusters in words and sentences, used with children from age 2 upwards; other tests by the same authors test auditory skills (from age 3 upwards) and auditory discrimination (from age 4 upwards).

Illinois Test of Psycholinguistic Abilities (revised edn.) (ITPA), by S. A. Kirk, J. J. McCarthy and W. D. Kirk, is a diagnostic test (containing 12 subtests) which evaluates the ability of children aged 2 to 10 in terms of channels of communication (auditory-vocal and visual-motor), psycholinguistic processes (receptive, organizing, and expressive), and levels of organization (automatic and representative) (see also, p. 64).

Language Assessment, Remediation and Screening Procedure (LARSP), by D. Crystal, P. Fletcher and M. Garman, is a method of grammatical analysis which produces a profile description of a child or adult language sample, as the basis for clinical assessment and remediation.

Merrill-Palmer Pre-School Performance Tests, by R. Stutsman, constitutes a series of 19 tests designed to assess the general behavioural performance of children between 1½ and 5 years.

Minnesota Test for Differential Diagnosis of Aphasia, by H. Schuell, is a series of tests aimed at assessing language disturbance in adult aphasics; it contains five sections: auditory disturbance, visual and reading disturbance, speech and language disturbance, visual motor and writing disturbance and disturbances of numerical relations and arithmetical processes.

Northwest Syntax Screening Test, by L. L. Lee, provides a quick estimate of receptive and expressive use of a series of syntactic structures by children between 3 and 8.

Peabody Picture Vocabulary Test, by L. M. Dunn, is a graded series of 150 plates, each containing 4 pictures; a stimulus word is used to elicit the child's ability to point to the correct picture; used for children from age 2½ in most categories of handicap.

Phonological Assessment of Child Speech (PACS), by P. Grunwell, is a set of procedures for analysing in depth the difficulties children have with consonants and consonant clusters; it contains a developmental dimension, and gives a series of profiles that can be used for assessment and remediation.

Porch Index of Communicative Ability (PICA), by B. E. Porch, contains a series of 18 tests aimed at evaluating communicative ability (verbal, gestural, graphic) in aphasic adults; responses are scored using a multidimensional system (one in which a patient's response is simultaneously evaluated along several dimensions). (A children's version is also in experimental use.)

Profile of Phonology (PROPH), by D. Crystal & P. Fletcher, is a profile description of English vowels, consonants, and consonant clusters, which classifies normal and abnormal productions according to general phonetic principles.

Profile in Semantics (PRISM), by D. Crystal, is a two-part profile description of lexical and grammatical aspects of semantic structure; *PRISM-L* provides a classification of the vocabulary of language samples, organized partly in developmental terms; *PRISM-G* describes the range of meanings expressed by grammatical structures, related to the stages of development recognised on LARSP (see above).

Prosody Profile (PROP), by D. Crystal, is a profile description of the main aspects of intonational structure, graded developmentally.

Renfrew Language Attainment Scales are a series of four tests devised by Catherine Renfrew for use with young children; the *Articulation attainment test* estimates the use of English consonants, for children between 3 and 6; *The Bus Story* is a test of continuous speech, between 3 and 8; the *Word-finding vocabulary scale* assesses the child's ability to use words (3-8 yrs); the *Picture vocabulary test* assesses word recognition using pictures.

Reynell Developmental Language Scales (revised edn.), by Joan Reynell, contains scales for the separate assessment of expressive language and verbal comprehension for children between 1½ and 6 years.

Sentence Comprehension Test, by K. Wheldall, P. Mittler & A. Hobsbaum, provides an assessment of several aspects of receptive grammatical ability; it is designed for children between 3 and 5 years.

Stanford-Binet Intelligence Scale, revised by L. M. Terman and M. A. Merrill (revised 1960 version), assesses general intelligence on a range of verbal and nonverbal tasks from 2 years to adulthood.

Stycar Tests, by Mary Sheridan, are a series of tests on vision, hearing and language for children between 6 months and 7 years.

Test for the Auditory Comprehension of Language (TACL), by E. Carrow Woolfolk, is an assessment of receptive language, covering aspects of vocabulary, morphology, and syntax; designed for children between 3 and 6; there is an associated screening test.

Test for the Reception of Grammar (TROG), by D. Bishop, assesses the comprehension of a range of grammatical structures in children aged between 4 and 13.

Token Test (TT), by E. De Renzi and L. A. Vignolo is a battery of tests designed to identify deficits in the abilities of adult aphasic patients; the patient is instructed to manipulate a series of coloured tokens according to various commands, which increase in complexity. A later version, known as the *Reporter's Test (RT)* is a development of the expressive side of the test.

Wechsler Intelligence Scale for Children (revised) (WISC) by D. Wechsler, contains 5 verbal and 5 performance tests for children between 6½ and 16½. The *Wechsler Preschool and Primary Scale of Intelligence (WPPSI)* contains 5 verbal and 5 performance subtests aimed at children in the 4–6½ year range. The *Wechsler Adult Intelligence Scale (WAIS)* consists of 6 verbal and 5 performance subtests, and is used with people over the age of 16.

Wepman Auditory Discrimination Test, by J. Wepman, is a screening test for children aged between 5 and 8, in which a child has to state whether pairs of words are the same or different.

Further reading

Political background

Bullock Report (1975): *A language for life*. (London, HMSO)

Court Report (1976): *Fit for the future*. Report of the Committee on Child Health Services. (London, HMSO)

Fish Report (1985): *Educational opportunities for all?* (London, HMSO)

Halsbury Report (1975): Report of the Committee of Inquiry into pay and related conditions of service of the professions supplementary to medicine and speech therapists. (London, HMSO)

Quirk Report (1972): *Speech therapy services*. (London, HMSO)

Swann Report (1985): *Education for all* (London, HMSO)

Warnock Report (1978): *Special educational needs*. Report of the Committee of Inquiry into the education of handicapped children and young people. (London, HMSO)

Biological and medical background

Espir, M. L. E. and Rose, C. (1976): *The basic neurology of speech*. 2nd edn. (Oxford, Blackwell)

Green, J. H. (1972): *An introduction to human physiology*. 3rd edn. (London, OUP)

Horrobin, D. F. (1968): *Medical physiology and biochemistry*. (London, Edward Arnold)

Hinchcliffe, R. and Harrison, D. (1976): *Scientific foundations of otolaryngology*. (London, Heinemann)

Illingworth, R. S. (1972): *The development of the infant and young child*. (London, Churchill Livingstone)

Macleod, J. (ed.) (1974): *Davidson's principles and practice of medicine*, 11th edn. (London, Churchill Livingstone)

Mitchell, G. A. G. (1973): *The essentials of neuroanatomy*. (London, Churchill Livingstone)

Romanes, G. (ed.) (1972): *Cunningham's manual of practical anatomy*, vol. 3, *Head, neck and brain*. 11th edn. (London, OUP)

Young, J. Z. (1971): *An introduction to the study of man*. (Oxford, Clarendon Press)

Psychology background

Aitchison, J. (1987): *Words in the mind: an introduction to the mental lexicon.* (Oxford, Blackwell)

Argyle, M. (1988): *Bodily communication.* 2nd edn. (London, Methuen)

Garnham, A. (1985): *Psycholinguistics: central topics.* (London, Methuen)

Harris, M. & Coltheart, M. (1986): *Language processing in children and adults.* (London, Routledge & Kegan Paul)

Hilgard, E. R., Atkinson, R. C. and Atkinson, R. L. (1975): *Introduction to psychology.* 6th edn. (New York, Harcourt Brace Jovanovich)

Milner, G. B. (1970): *Physiological psychology.* (New York, Holt, Rinehart & Winston)

Mittler, P. (1970): *The psychological assessment of mental and physical handicaps.* (London, Methuen)

Mussen, P. H., Conger, J. J. and Kagan, J. (1969): *Child development and personality.* 3rd edn. (New York, Harper & Row)

Language and linguistics background

Bolinger, D. L. and Sears, D. A. (1981): *Aspects of language.* 3rd edn. (New York, Harcourt Brace Jovanovich)

Cherry, C. (1961): *On human communication.* (New York, Science Editions)

Clark, E. and Clark, H. H. (1977): *Psychology and language, an introduction to psycholinguistics.* (New York, Harcourt Brace Jovanovich)

Cruttenden, A. (1979): *Language in infancy and childhood.* (Manchester, Manchester University Press)

Crystal, D. (1984): *Linguistic encounters with language handicap.* (Oxford, Blackwell)

Crystal, D. (1985): *Linguistics.* 2nd edn. (Harmondsworth, Penguin)

Crystal, D. (1981/7): *Clinical linguistics.* (Vienna, Springer; London, Edward Arnold)

Dale, P. S. (1976): *Language development: structure and function.* 2nd edn. (Hinsdale, Ill., Dryden Press)

Denes, P. B. and Pinson, E. N. (1973): *The speech chain: the physics and biology of spoken language.* (New York, Anchor Books)

Fry, D. B. (1977): *Homo loquens: man as a talking animal.* (Cambridge, CUP)

Grunwell, P. (1987): *Clinical phonology.* 2nd edn. (London, Croom Helm)

O'Connor, J. D. (1973): *Phonetics.* (Harmondsworth, Penguin)

Palmer, F. R. (1984): *Grammar.* 2nd edn. (Harmondsworth, Penguin)

Lenneberg, E. H. (1967): *Biological foundations of language.* (New York, Wiley)

Language pathology background
Aram, D. M. and Nation, J. E. (1982): *Child language disorders.* (St. Louis, Mosby)
Baken, R. J. (1987): *Clinical measurement of speech and voice.* (Boston, College-Hill Press)
Bamford, J. and Saunders, E. (1985): *Hearing impairment, auditory perception and language disability.* (London, Edward Arnold)
Beasley, D. S. and Davis, G. A. (1981): *Aging: communication process and disorders.* (New York, Grune and Stratton)
Bloom, L. and Lahey, M. (1978): *Language development and language disorders.* (New York, Wiley)
Bryant, P. and Bradley, L. (1985): *Children's reading problems: psychology and education.* (Oxford, Blackwell)
Carrow-Woolfolk, E. and Lynch, J. I. (1982): *An integrative approach to language disorders in children.* (New York, Grune and Stratton)
Darley, F. and Spriestersbach, D. (1978): *Diagnostic methods in speech pathology.* 2nd edn. (New York, Harper & Row)
Davis, H. S. and Silverman, S. (eds.) (1970): *Hearing and deafness.* 3rd edn. (New York, Holt Rinehart & Winston)
Gillham, B. (ed.) (1986): *Handicapping conditions in children.* (London, Croom Helm)
Luchsinger, R. and Arnold, G. E. (1965): *Voice—speech—language.* (London, Constable)
Miles, T. R. and Miles, E. (1983): *Help for dyslexic children.* (London, Methuen)
Morley, M. (1972): *The development and disorders of speech in childhood.* 3rd edn. (London, Churchill Livingstone)
Müller, D. J., Munro, S. M. and Code, C. (1981): *Language assessment for remediation.* (London, Croom Helm)
Nation, J. E. and Aram, D. M. (1984): *Diagnosis of speech and language disorders.* 2nd edn. (St. Louis, Mosby)
Nicolosi, L., Harryman, E. and Kresheck, J. (1978): *Terminology of communication disorders.* (Baltimore, Williams & Wilkins)
Perkins, W. H. (1977): *Speech pathology: an applied behavioural science.* 2nd edn. (St. Louis, Mosby)
Rieber, R. W. & Brubaker, R. S. (eds.) (1966): *Speech pathology.* (Amsterdam, North-Holland)
Shames, G. H. and Wiig, E. H. (1984): *Human communication disorders: an introduction.* (Columbus, Merrill)
Snowling, M. J. (ed.) (1985): *Children's written language difficulties.* (Windsor, NFER-Nelson)
Thomson, M. (1984): *Developmental dyslexia.* (London, Edward Arnold)
Travis, L. E. (ed.) (1971): *Handbook of speech pathology.* 2nd edn. (New York, Appleton-Century-Crofts)
Warner, J. A. W., Byers Brown, B. and McCartney, E. (1984): *Speech*

218   *Introduction to language pathology*

therapy: a clinical companion. (Manchester, Manchester University Press)

Webster, A. and McConnell, C. (1987): *Special needs in ordinary schools.* (London, Cassell)

Williams, P. (ed.) (1988): *A glossary of special education.* (Milton Keynes, Open University Press)

Wren, C. T. (1983): *Language learning disabilities: diagnosis and remediation.* (Rockville, Aspen Systems)

Yule, W. and Rutter, M. (1987): *Language development and disorders.* (London, Mac Keith Press)

Index of names

Index of subjects

aversion therapy 28
axon 72

bar 112
basal ganglia 79, 156
basilar membrane 117–18
behaviour 27–8, 69, 198–9
  modification 28
  therapy 27–8
behaviourism 27
bilateral 133, 156, 189–90
bilingualism 207–8
binaural 133
biotic 21
blocking 167–8
blood supply 86–8
Boston Diagnostic Aphasia
    Examination 210
brain 55, 62–72, 74–93, 141–2, 148–9,
    157, 171, 173
  , mid- 79
  , split- 92
  stem 75, 79
British Ability Scales 210
British Deaf Association 135
British Journal of Disorders of
    Communication 2
British Picture Vocabulary Scale 210
British Sign Language 33, 135
bulbar palsy 89

carcinoma 107, 177
caseload 30–31
CAT scanning 88
central pathologies 140–65
cerebellum 75, 79, 156
cerebrum 75–7
chemotherapy 69
Child Language Teaching and
    Therapy 198, 209
chimpanzees 63
choanae 107
circle of Willis 86–8
circumlocution 145, 167
clause 44, 66
cleft palate, *see* palate
Clinical Language Intervention
    Programme (CLIP) 210–11
clinical linguistics 198–206
  diagnosis in 204–6
Clinical Linguistics & Phonetics 198, 199
cluttering 173
cochlea 117–19, 131, 133
cochlear duct 117–18

cochlear implanting 119, 199
cocktail party phenomenon 121
cognition 64–5, 161–2
College of Speech Therapists 2, 4
Coloured Progressive Matrices 211
communication 7, 33
  aids 208–9
  , attitude to 11, 169–70, 179
  chain 54–121, 122, 150–51
  v. language 33–7
  modes 7, 124, 146–7
community quality 36
compensation 123, 180
competence 38
comprehension 85, 142–4, 148, 187
compulsion 68
computer-aided interaction 209
conditions
  , communicative 60
  , etiological 24
conduction
  ,air v. bone 113–14, 131
conductive 131
congenital 21, 50, 107–8, 119, 133–4, 161
connector 44
consonant 99, 101, 103–5, 111–12, 154,
    182–6
  clusters 185–7
  , types of 103–5
contact ulcers 107–8, 177–8
contralaterality 81, 84
contrasts 185–6
conversational skills 200–2
conversion
  aphonia 178–9
  reactions 68
corpus callosum 79, 90, 148
cortex 79–93
  , motor 81, 88–9
  , sensory 83
  , sub- 90
critical period 51–2, 147
cued speech 135
CVA 86–8, 143, 146
cycle 110

damped 110
deaf
  -blind 8
  , teacher of the 125, 134
deafish 137
deafness 6–7, 26, 123, 129–40, 162
  , pure word 148
  , types of 131–4

psychosis 67–9
psychosomatic 69
psychotherapy 69–70, 157
psychotic 68–9
puberphonia 176
pure word deafness 148, 151–2
pyramidal tracts 81

quadrantic 85
Quirk Report 2, 30–31, 193–4, 197

reading 6–7, 84, 92, 146–7, 152, 206
recall 64
reception 55–7, 61, 64, 122–3, 129–40,
   142, 145–6, 150–51, 161–2
recognition 64, 120, 150–51
recording 30–31
recurrent laryngeal nerve 98, 178
   palsy 107–8
redintegration 64
referral 23
reflex 35, 120
relearning 64
Renfrew Tests 213
repetition 166, 168
Reporter's Test (RT) 213
resonance 174–80
resonate 110
resonators 99
respiratory cycle 95
Reynell Scales 213
rhinology 106
rhythm 154, 161–2, 166–8
roll 103–5
rounding 101, 103–5
round window 117
Royal National Institute for the Deaf 129
rules 37–40

sampling 29, 163
scala tympani 117–18
scala vestibuli 117–18
schizophrenia 68–9, 157–9, 200
schools 128, 130
scotoma 85
segmental 103–5
semantic-pragmatic disorder 200
semantics 41, 45–7, 124–6, 144, 162,
   164–5, 199
semicircular canals 116–17
semiotics 7–8
senescence 22, 177
senility 68
sensorineural 131

sensory 72, 81–3, 88–9, 123, 124–5, 131,
   142
sentence 44
   length 44–5
   structure 44
Sentence Comprehension Test 213
sequencing 64, 157, 159
signs 18, 23–6, 135–6
sinusitis 106
sinusoidal 110
sociolinguistics 47, 129, 180
somatic 74
somatotherapy 69
sone 114
sound pressure level 112
spastic dysarthria 156
special needs 207
spectrogram 111–12
spectrum 111
speech 6–8, 10, 124–6
   chain 54
   therapy 1–6, 70, 125, 193–4, 195–7,
      198, 203–6
spiral ligament 117–18
stammering, *see* stuttering
Stanford-Binet Scale 213
stapedectomy 119
stapes 116
stenosis 86
stereotype 137, 147, 157, 160
stridor 175
stroke 9, 13, 17, 26, 86–8, 194
structural 106, 180
stuttering 8, 23, 58, 123, 155, 166–73,
   204
   , theories of 170–72
   , types of 170
Stycar Tests 213
subject 44, 45, 66
submucous 189
substitution 126–7, 144, 184–6
sub-titling 208
sulcus 79–84
symbolic 124, 140–41, 161–2
symptoms 18, 23–6
synapse 73
synchronic 50, 60
synonymy 45
syntax 43
   , developmental 52

tactile 7
tape-repeater 31
team approach 195, 207